IS MY HORSE IN PAIN?

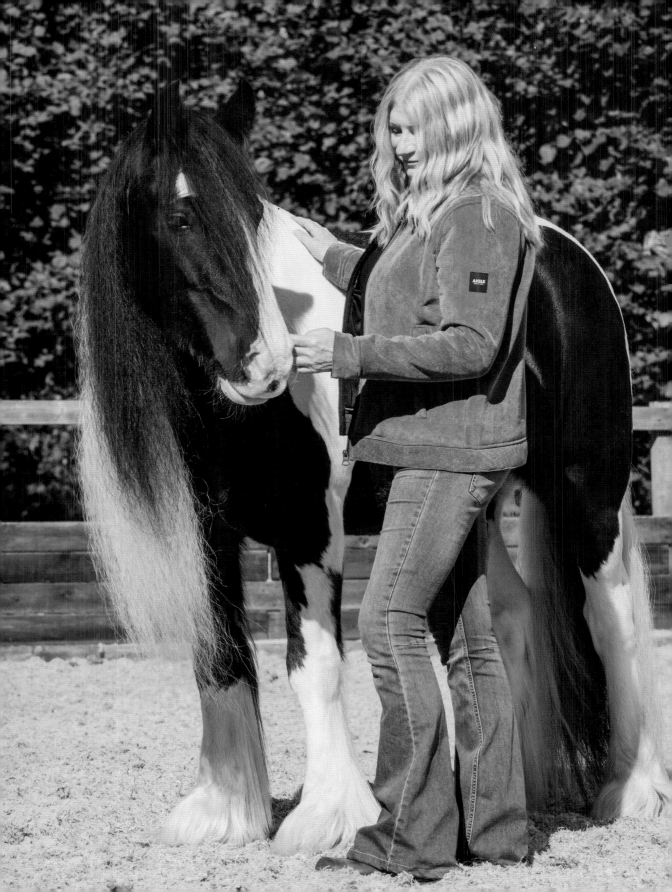

IS MY HORSE IN PAIN?

A Guide to Assessing and Improving Your Horse's Musculoskeletal Health and Performance

ANGELA HALL

J.A. ALLEN

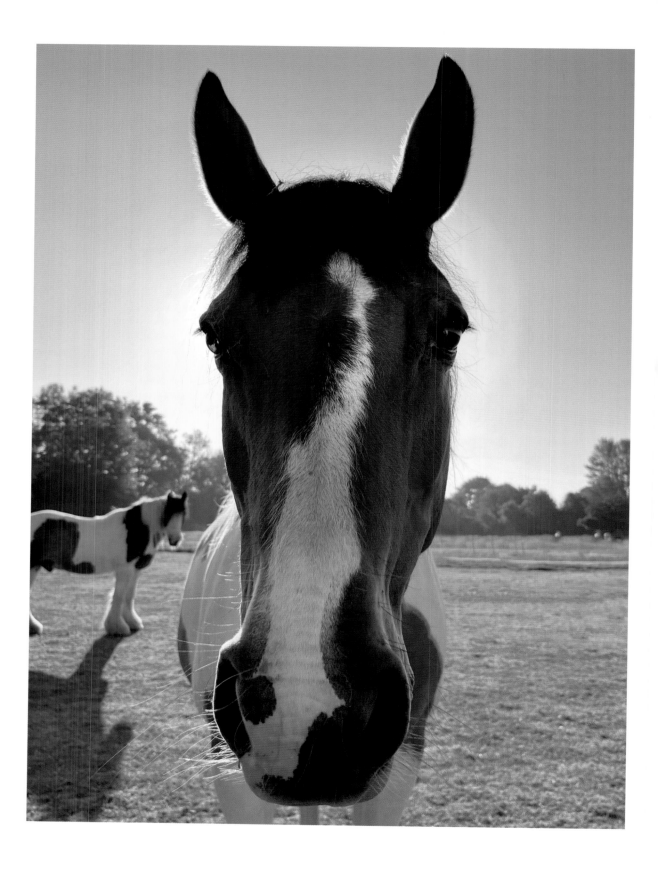

Contents

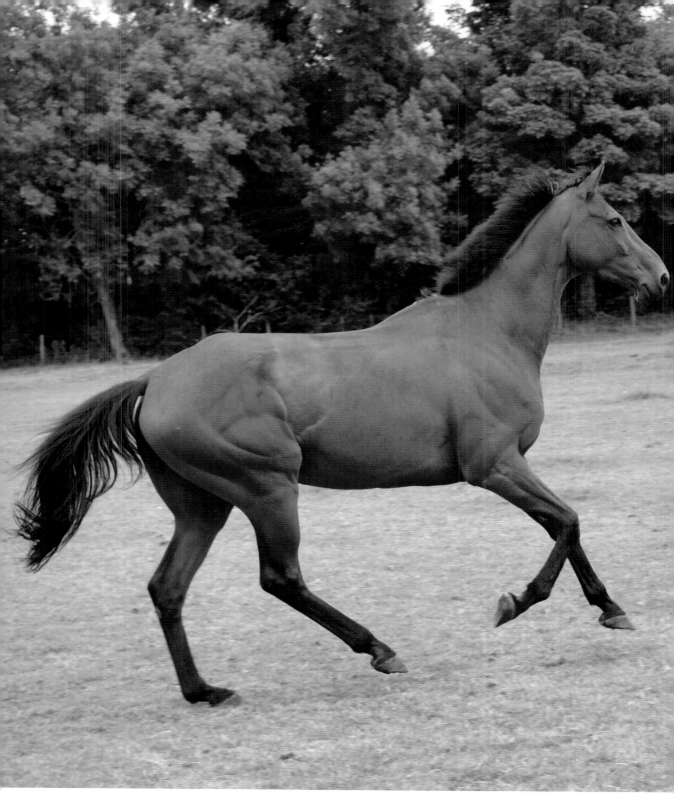

My gentle ex-racehorse Joe, with a newfound love for playing in the field, which was an entirely novel experience for him after race training; he quickly learned to appreciate the liberating feeling it brought.

Preface

In the vast tapestry of the animal kingdom, there is one creature that has captivated our imagination, stirred our souls, and stood beside us throughout the ages – the horse. Majestic and powerful, the horse has been our loyal companion, helping us forge empires, explore new lands and gallop towards the horizon of our dreams. Yet, in our quest to harness their incredible strength and beauty, we must also examine the profound responsibility of caretakers to ensure their health and wellbeing.

Within the realm of horsemanship, it becomes essential to develop a deep understanding of the horse, to perceive the subtle nuances hidden beneath their gentleness and within the rhythm of their movements. It is through this understanding that we can truly connect with them on a profound level, nurturing their physical and emotional wellbeing while unlocking their full potential.

The journey to comprehend and fully meet the needs of our equine companions is an ongoing exploration guided by ever-evolving research, a journey that requires dedication, empathy, and a ceaseless thirst for knowledge. As equestrians, in whatever capacity we operate, it is our duty to ensure that our horses thrive in an environment that promotes their overall peace and comfort.

Within the pages of *Is My Horse in Pain?*, we embark on a transformative expedition into the heart of equine wellness, drawing upon a wealth of expert insight, practical experience, and scientific knowledge. This book serves as a compass, guiding us through the labyrinthine pathways of equine understanding, anatomy, physiology, conformation and biomechanics and much more; leading to the core of the book, equine 'manual' therapy and correct supportive exercise to explore the ways in which we can alleviate pain and discomfort, restore harmony and optimise our horses' wellbeing and performance.

I understand the challenges you face in the equine world, but if you follow my guidance in this book, which is presented in a manner that is accessible and easy to comprehend, you will make great progress. Remember that change takes time, so you must be patient. By being flexible and open to new ideas, you are starting to charter a new course, and I wish you great success.

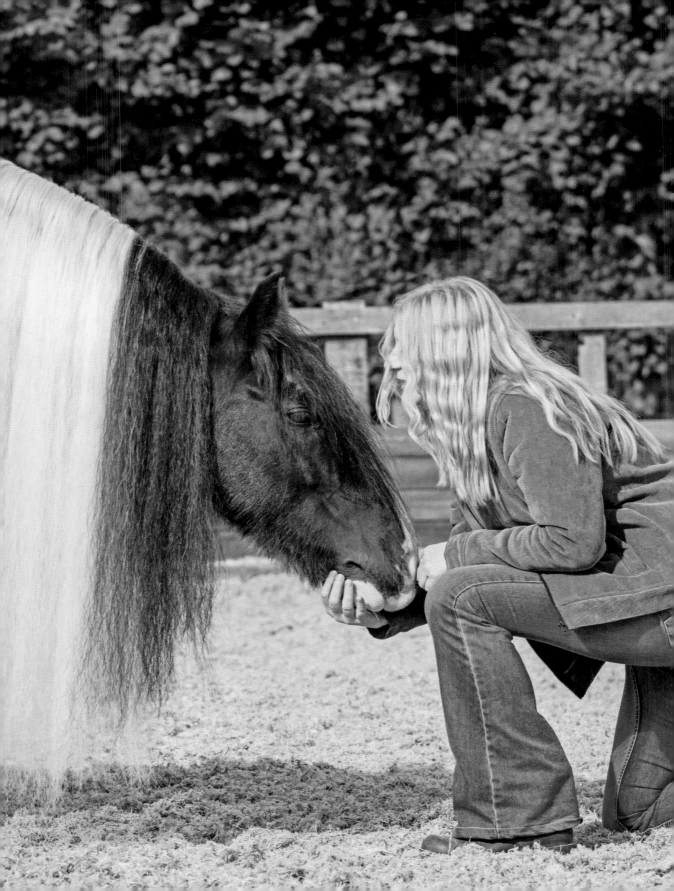

PART I – UNDERSTANDING

CHAPTER I

Understanding and Managing Your Horse to Avoid Pain and Injury

It is my intention to provide valuable information on how to develop a deeper understanding of horses and their needs, as well as effective practices for managing them to prevent pain and injury. I would never underestimate the knowledge and experience of any equestrian; I aim for you to think differently about your horse and your relationship with it, adopting the principles that I use, with success, when working with horses of all disciplines on a worldwide scale. I will help you find anything that affects your horse's wellbeing, safety and opportunities for success.

The horse's mind, body and spirit are all connected – functionally, neurologically and metabolically; therefore, adopting an holistic approach to understanding and managing your horse can have a distinct impact on its health, welfare and performance. All of this underpins the core concept of this book, which is to learn how to accurately apply equine manual therapy to your horse alongside correct supportive exercise.

Many books – such as those focusing on becoming a better rider – cover specific aspects of horse management. These are well written and informative about muscle function, biomechanics, training methods and how a horse and rider can improve performance. Nonetheless, they frequently fail to consider the entire horse and how its mind, body and spirit connections underpin everything. If, for example, the horse's physical health is impaired due to pain from conditions such as osteoarthritis or gastric ulcers, it will be unable to perform specific movements that the owner may read about in a book but wonder why the horse cannot do as the book suggests. This can occur if the horse's emotional and physical health has been compromised. You must understand the importance of your management functions and consider them along with the whole horse and how each intertwines with the other, significantly impacting the horse's health, welfare and performance.

We must explore particular elements of horse management before we embark on the book's core topic, manual therapy and how and when you can apply it correctly to your horse. Horse management encompasses everything involved in caring for a horse and I will include specifics that affect a horse's musculoskeletal health directly or indirectly. Correct horse management is crucial, because it provides the necessary knowledge to ensure that a horse's basic needs are met, which is fundamental to its overall health and welfare. For example, if a horse is fed incorrectly, it may not receive the necessary nutrients for muscle growth and performance, leading to health problems and training and development issues.

You may already be very experienced in horse management; my aim is not to question that but to highlight some specific aspects that will further establish a strong foundation for successful training and manual therapy with benefits your horse will reap.

Understanding Equine Behaviour and Survival Instincts

Understanding equine behaviour and its unpredictable nature can be complex. It is essential that we try to understand their world and how we can best accommodate and manage them in ours to coexist in harmony. Humans can affect horses positively or negatively, as their behaviour, performance, diseases and injuries reflect our management and expectations. To understand horses, we must stop, observe, and listen to them as they express their feelings through behaviour, body language, reluctance to work, performance, lameness and illness. If a horse cannot or does not do what we ask, the reasons are usually simple: it does not understand, is not physically capable, or is in pain. Emotional disturbances can also affect the physical body, as seen in human medicine; this applies to horses too.

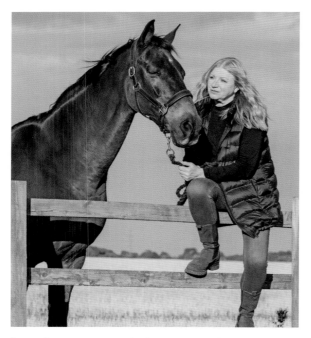

By embracing a more holistic approach, you can identify areas where your management could be improved to enrich your horse's overall health and wellbeing and strengthen your bond. For horses to thrive mentally and physically, they require a sense of harmony.

THE PREY ANIMAL

All animals have instincts that make them either prey or predator. Horses are highly instinctive prey animals that require a sense of safety to thrive. In herd groups, horses feel secure and protected. When they sense danger, they switch to instinctive behaviour such as 'fight or flight'. Horses are always on guard, so it is important to understand and assist them rather than blame them when they exhibit normal behaviour, such as shying at objects or becoming restless on a hack.

Being quietly confident and taking time around the horse can help maintain its relaxation and reduce stress hormone levels. An increase in cortisol is natural in response to episodes of acute stress, but when raised daily due to chronic stress from management or the environment, it harms the horse. Lack of turnout, isolation, inability to roll and heavy training schedules are all management factors that can increase stress hormone levels, leading to illness, impaired performance and musculoskeletal problems, including Cushing's disease and colic.

High cortisol levels can lead to an uncomfortable frame in the horse, including a high head carriage and a hollow back, causing tension in both body and mind. This posture triggers the horse's natural 'flight' response, making it more challenging to handle and more likely to take flight. Fear can be seen in the horse's eyes when the sclera (white of the eye) is visible in extreme circumstances.

This horse should be comforted – not punished – and encouraged to cease moving in this hollow frame. Training aids will also injure the horse in this frame, as it sets itself against them. Instead, evaluate the horse's management, environment and treatment to make it more comfortable and less 'high-alert' and start a programme of supportive correct exercise to improve its frame, as shown in Chapter 8.

Horses on professional yards, especially in race training, often have a high head carriage and hollow back. Group schooling in this way may not suit all horses, due to their diverse personalities. Even hacking with a spooky horse can transfer negative en-

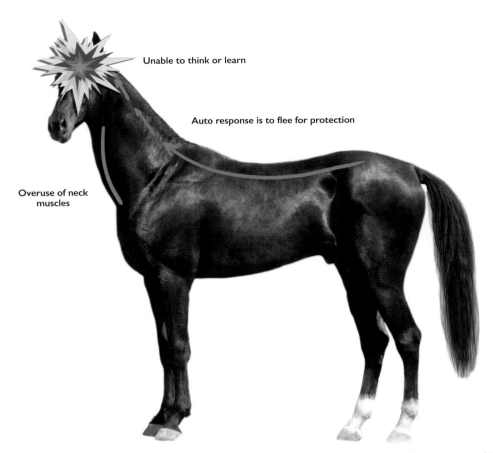

Unable to think or learn

Auto response is to flee for protection

Overuse of neck muscles

This horse exhibits signs of mental imbalance, as indicated by its high head carriage, which impairs its ability to think and learn effectively. Additionally, its hollow back is an instinctive reaction triggered by the urge to flee for protection. The horse's excessive use of its neck is apparent from the pronounced muscle development on the underside, resulting from holding its head too high too frequently.

ergy to other horses. Personalised training is essential for each horse's benefit. Owners have a responsibility to understand their horses and make management decisions to help them feel comfortable and safe. Punishing horses for exhibiting natural behaviour is not acceptable.

These horses will benefit from manual therapy, as it reduces cortisol levels by inducing the parasympathetic nervous system, which helps with body posture and movement patterns as the horse relaxes and releases tension. The techniques to perform are those in the maintenance category shown in Chapter 7.

PREY DEFENCE AND LAMENESS DETECTION

Lameness can start anywhere in the body and may not be obvious because horses are programmed to hide their vulnerabilities to evade predators by displaying 'prey defence'. Very often, I see horses in which the lameness has usually reached the stage where the horse can no longer disguise it; this makes it more challenging to diagnose by the veterinarian and to treat.

Subtle signs that something is not right should be addressed before the situation worsens. These can often be discovered during manual therapy sessions as issues in the upper body – particularly the neck, shoulders, back, and sacroiliac region – and can eventually present as limb lameness. The appropriate techniques for this purpose belong to the maintenance category.

Communicating with the Horse

It is important to remember when communicating with horses that they rely heavily on body language and non-verbal cues. Horses are incredibly sensitive to the energy and emotions of the people around them, so it is essential to remain calm, clear and consistent in your movements and demeanour when interacting with them.

Additionally, it is crucial to take the time to learn and understand your horse's body language and communication methods so that you can effectively communicate with them and build a trusting relationship. If you fail to understand the true meaning of them, it can lead to conflict in your relationship.

Working with numerous horses has taught me that peaceful people always get better results from their horses. To optimise the effectiveness of your manual therapy sessions with your horse, it is best to schedule them during quiet periods in the yard and ensure you are not in a hurry or experiencing high energy levels. It is also important to maintain a calm and deliberate approach when interacting with the horse – moving and speaking slowly. Remember that horses can hear a wider range of frequencies than humans, so try to be aware of any sounds in their surroundings that you may not perceive but they will.

Horses possess a distinct energy, which becomes more apparent in settings where they are employed for therapeutic purposes. Through my experiences, I have learned that being in a horse's presence leads to a mutual exchange of energy. When interacting with a calm and composed horse, I feel at peace as well. Conversely, if I work with a horse that is anxious or has suffered abuse, I take on their feelings of distress. This ability to attune to horses allows me to better comprehend and connect with them, which brings a special quality to the therapy I provide.

THE HUMAN–HORSE RELATIONSHIP

The human–horse relationship is unique and special and has evolved over thousands of years. Once the relationship with your horse generates confidence, it can be further enhanced with manual therapy, walking together, or simply hanging out. It is not always about riding and competing with the horse; this can indicate the horse becoming machine-like, especially if it is overdone. A horse is a living, thinking, sentient being, which must be respected as a majestic creature and not a possession; after all, the horse was

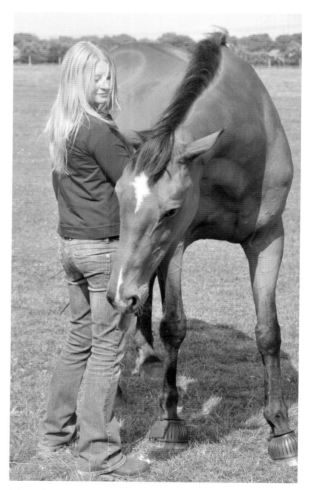

I loved spending time with my gorgeous thoroughbred horse Shamus, who reached 28 years – just being with him, grooming, massaging and exchanging energy. People did not understand why I did not always ride him. I was fulfilled by being in his presence, as was he. My deep and unique relationship with my horse did not need an explanation to anyone.

never designed to be ridden.

Owning a horse is not about being the alpha or being led by peer pressure; it is about confidence, trust, understanding, respect, tolerance and kindness. Equestrians who exhibit these positive traits have better relationships with their horses; the horse becomes a faithful companion willing to please, often excelling in their equestrian discipline because it is comfortable, happier and more likely to stay pain and injury-free by being trained correctly and sympathetically.

If you are struggling to comprehend your horse, or the relationship between you two is not proving beneficial, you should seek assistance from a qualified and respected equine behaviour professional. Additionally, as an owner, there are things you can do to strengthen the bond with your horse – such as spending quality time together grooming, performing manual therapy and hand grazing. The horse and the human should feel secure and comfortable in each other's company. If the horse has had unpleasant experiences, bonding and desensitisation exercises can help alleviate their response to past traumas. It is crucial to persist and work with the horse instead of rejecting it due to misunderstood behaviour, which is regrettably all too common in the industry.

Meeting the Horse's Basic Needs

Managing a horse and meeting its basic needs is essential for the animal's physical and mental wellbeing. Horses are large, complex animals that require a significant amount of care and attention to remain healthy and happy. Proper management includes providing the horse with adequate food and water, shelter, correct exercise, reducing its stress levels and much more. By meeting these basic needs, horse owners can help prevent health problems and ensure their horse has a good quality of life. Additionally, a well-managed horse is likelier to perform better in various activities, such as ridden work or competition, and develop a strong bond with its owner or handler.

This is a significant responsibility that requires a commitment to the animal's care and wellbeing. Here are some aspects that, if not managed correctly, can lead to major health problems.

GRAZING

Horses should graze for around fifteen hours daily, as they only have small stomachs and therefore need regular sustenance. Sadly, they often go without food for long periods in their stables, day and night, which can lead to negative behaviours from the horse. It is best to provide ad-lib forage when possible. They also need to browse for roots, bark and other plants for essential nutrients. Zoopharmacognosy shows that horses self-select plants to address various physical and psychological conditions; as a Master in Herbology, I am keenly interested in natural medicine for horses.

Recent research found that milk thistle causes health benefits to horses, including anti-inflammatory and antioxidant properties. Studies also show that exercise increases cortisol, with peak levels observed at fifteen to thirty minutes after exercise; when horses were supplemented with milk thistle, they had a significantly lower increase in cortisol after fifteen minutes of exercise. For such reasons, I include natural medicine for horses in my range of online courses, because I know the profound benefits of it.

Pasture management is crucial to maintain quality grazing, and a stocking rate of one horse per two acres is recommended. Overstocking can lead to land damage and nutritional deficiencies for the horse. Not fulfilling the horse's natural grazing and browsing needs can cause emotional and physical problems.

To ensure nutrient quality, it is recommended to have an agronomist test your horse's grazing and all forage. Providing a diet of grass, forage, concentrated feed, balancers, supplements, fruits, vegetables, and treats is not advisable. It is essential to confirm the nutrient content of the base diet of grass and forage before adding any additional components, as over-supplementation can lead to toxicity, bone, and muscle damage.

FEEDING AND NUTRITION

Feeding horses does not have to be complicated. The horse's digestive system is simple and relies on forage for gut health. For most performance horses, forage alone provides sufficient energy. Linseed oil can be an alternative for controlled energy release. Overfeeding grain disrupts the microbiome, causing health issues like colic, hindgut acidosis, and bone/muscle conditions. If the horse shows abdominal discomfort during manual therapy, reconsider its diet. Digestive system disruption affects performance and mental ability and can be linked to headshaking. Starch-rich diets are known to contribute to behavioural problems.

HAY NET FEEDING

Italian researchers (Raspa *et al*, March 2021) studied the effects of hay net feeding on the horse's back, neck and jaw angles. Six horses were observed eating from three positions: ground, knee-level and high hay net. Using geometric morphometrics, the researchers found that the low hay net position resulted in a natural back position with elongated muscles, while the higher hay net position shortened the muscles. As the neck raised, the jawline-neck angle closed, creating

unnatural eating angles. The researchers emphasised the importance of understanding the body positions created by hay nets and the safety implications of height positioning.

It is beneficial to massage your horses throughout their neck and back if they are feeding from hay nets, especially if these are placed at a higher level. Even when they are placed at the lower level, due to the horse grasping and tearing at the contents of the hay net, I see increased tension in the face, head and neck muscles of these horses compared to those fed from the ground without a hay net.

DRINKING WATER

Water is essential for horses – to regulate body temperature, transport compounds and lubricate joints. A horse's water consumption varies with their feed moisture, workload and climate, but on average, a 500kg (1,102lb) horse in work should drink around 50 litres of water daily, or 10 litres per 100kg (220lb) of weight. Horses without access to grazing need more water due to the higher dry feed intake. If a horse does not consume enough water, it can dehydrate, negatively affecting its health and performance.

Automatic water feeders should be regularly cleaned and fitted with water gauges, and tubs should be managed based on water content. Even if a horse does not consume its recommended daily intake, it still needs access to that amount.

HEALTH CARE

I firmly believe that everyone who cares for a horse should learn equine first aid, because they are often the first to discover an injury and are required to act. My training company offers online equine first aid training for horse owners whereby other useful skills can also be learned, such as correctly taking the horse's vital signs, temperature, pulse and respiration. I recommend that the horse's vital signs are taken weekly to monitor responses to training and its general health, as they are the primary indicator of health status. This is a key aspect of horse ownership that is often overlooked.

Farriery and dental care should be done on a cycle to align with changes in the foot and oral cavity; six-weekly intervals are recommended for farriery and six monthly for dental care.

TACK AND TRAINING AIDS

Tack and training aids can cause many performance limitations and injuries for horses. I have witnessed many failings due to incorrect bridle fit, nosebands and especially flash nosebands being tied too tightly,

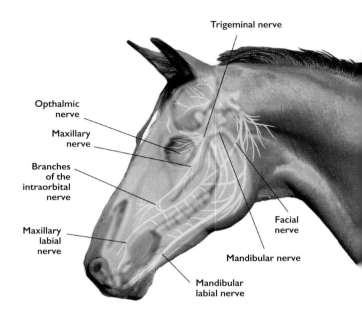

The facial nerves are located just below the skin and can be affected by pressure exerted by bridles and headcollars. This can interrupt the transmission of messages from the brain to the face and lead to significant discomfort for horses. The use of tight nosebands and flash nosebands can be particularly harmful and should be avoided.

the wrong bit and incorrect saddle and girth fit. As a rule, the simpler the equipment, the better. The tack must fit well and be comfortable. Placing tack over nerves, especially the facial cranial nerves, can be painful for the horse and hinder its performance.

Bespoke bits are necessary for horses, as their oral cavities and tongue sizes vary. Horses also have different preferences for pressure, either on the tongue or the bar. Wearing the correct bit is crucial, as it can affect a horse's performance and musculoskeletal health. The wrong bit can cause physical and behavioural problems, such as jaw pain, neck pain, shortened stride, reluctance to move forward and snatching at the bit.

I have seen saddles that damage the horse's muscles and spinal column, eventually rendering them unrideable. Bits that cut the horse's tongue, damage the hard palate, and in another instance, the horse's mouth, was tied so tightly in a flash noseband that it cut into the skin, and a sharp tooth severed the

> ## ★ TOP TIP
>
> I have observed that after a farrier visit, or when they are due for one, many horses exhibit suboptimal performance. This can be attributed to the impact on their posture caused by changes in the shape of their feet, which affect the fascia – the body's largest connective tissue. To mitigate these effects, it is advisable to incorporate your manual therapy in conjunction with farrier visits. A parallel can be drawn between this situation and how people experience postural changes when changing shoes. However, due to their quadrupedal nature, horses are more susceptible to significant alterations than bipedal humans.

horse's inner cheek, which became infected. This is purely due to bad management; we should not be seeing this, and there are no excuses.

Training aids that force horses into a frame can be damaging, causing pain, hairline fractures, and irreparable damage to muscles and bones; I have witnessed the effects during equine dissections. Overdeveloped neck muscles from tight side reins can lead to the inability of muscles to contract and relax correctly. Aids that connect the horse's hindquarters to the front end can be harmful if settings are too advanced, preventing the horse from developing self-carriage. Many traditional schooling styles, such as fiddling with the horse's mouth or pulling it into a frame with rigid hands, are not beneficial today. Horses ridden in a light, free frame appear to succeed with fewer injuries and can perform longer. Manual therapy and correct supportive exercise can help repair muscle damage and prevent recurring problems. Horses need their musculoskeletal systems maintained and cared for correctly to avoid pain and injury.

RIDER SUITABILITY

Many horse riders suffer from musculoskeletal injuries and long-term chronic conditions, which result in imbalances in the saddle. These generate through to the horse when riding, for which the horse will need to compensate, causing its own muscular tension and strain. I always advise my customers not to ride when they are in pain or after an injury. Instead, I recommend in-hand schooling, which can be beneficial and enjoyable for the horse. It gives the horse another focus and can relieve boredom.

Regular musculoskeletal therapy is essential for riders who plan to continue riding. Failing to do so will eventually cause the horse to reach a point where it can no longer compensate for the rider's issues. Even a small amount of damage over time can lead to the horse's body becoming crooked, resulting in biomechanical alterations that are challenging to re-align and often impossible to fix.

TRAVELLING

Travelling can be tough on horses due to the need to stabilise their heavy bodies during transit, causing fatigue and strain. Kinesio-taping and manual therapy can support horses that frequently travel for competitions. Journeys should be well planned and kept as infrequent and short as possible to reduce the impact on the horse's body.

A study by Dr G. Robert Colborne in 2021 found that horses use their legs as springs to dampen trailer vibrations while travelling. This can be very taxing on the horse's body, especially if they have pre-existing limb conditions such as osteoarthritis or tendon/ligament weakness. Rest and manual therapy are essential for the horse to recover after the journey.

SEASONAL CHANGES

Temperature, diet and exercise variations can heighten the risk of health issues such as respiratory infections, heat stress, dehydration, insect bites, allergies and fatigue from excessive schooling and competition. Owners should increase winter-feeding to maintain body weight and temperature while ensuring adequate hydration in summer. Exercise should be scheduled during cooler times in hot weather and continued on suitable surfaces in winter to keep the horse's systems active. Fluctuations in weight affect tack fit, which should be addressed directly instead of relying on using more or fewer saddle pads that may make the saddle too tight or unstable.

FINANCIAL

Owning a horse is a significant financial commitment, from the basic needs of stabling, feeding and farriery to added expenses such as tack, musculoskeletal therapy, travel costs and more. If owners suffer financially, their horses will suffer too. Sometimes, owners cannot afford diagnostic tests and treatments, leading to undiagnosed conditions. Unscheduled costs also occur when horses are unable to work due to injury or illness but still need to be stabled and fed. Some owners may rush their horse's return to work or retire them or even sell the horse by ruthlessly masking underlying problems with medication.

Educating horse owners is very beneficial to help identify issues early, preventing long-term damage to the horse and accumulating costs. Regular manual therapy helps detect warning signs that the horse's body is not right. My online training platform provides extensive learning for horse owners at reasonable fees.

The Horse's Environment

Horses, whether they are in paddocks or stables, require a safe and clean environment devoid of hazards and adverse weather conditions. Unfortunately, some facilities limit turnout during inclement weather, leading to extended periods of stabling in which horses experience physiological stagnation due to restricted movement and suffer from mental distress due to boredom. To address these concerns, it is essential to offer alternative turnout options, such as indoor arenas or outdoor sand enclosures, which contribute to the overall health and wellbeing of the horses. Moreover, when horses are compelled to spend prolonged periods in their stables, it is beneficial to provide deeper bedding, such as shavings or straw over rubber matting. This offers valuable support to the horses' limbs and facilitates the healing process, particularly for horses with weakened limbs or those undergoing rehabilitation from an injury.

Equine musculoskeletal injuries often stem from the horse's living environment. The confined space within stables can increase the risk of injuries during horse movement, entrances, exits and getting cast. Additionally, ground conditions play a role in injury

★ TOP TIP

While examining horses, I occasionally encounter cases with no major musculoskeletal issues, yet their performance seems diminished. In such situations, I assess their vital signs and frequently find abnormal temperature readings, which may indicate an underlying infection or illness. Neglecting these symptoms can have adverse effects on their performance and overall wellbeing. Therefore, it is vital to establish preventive measures that protect horses from diseases and infections, regularly monitor their vital signs, and promptly consult a veterinarian if any abnormalities arise.

occurrence, with concussive injuries more prevalent on firm ground during summer or winter and pulled muscles being a common concern on soft ground following heavy rain. To effectively prevent and manage such injuries, it is advisable to develop a seasonal plan incorporating routine check-ups by a musculoskeletal therapist, complemented by your manual therapy, and paying close attention to the horse's stabling, turn out areas and changes in ground surfaces can significantly contribute to injury prevention and management.

Disease control and biosecurity can be very poor among equestrians; there are no policies and practices in place at many establishments to avoid transmission, and very few have isolation areas or disease testing programmes in place. Horses travelling to compete are at a greater risk. Simple measures such as well-ventilated stabling, regular equipment cleaning and a walk-through foot bath for people and horses are a start. Horses should never share grooming equipment or tack under any circumstances, as these can harbour pathogens and pass on disease quickly.

The Horse's Emotional Wellbeing

The emotional wellbeing of a horse is crucial, as it directly affects its physical health. It is essential to pay close attention to any changes in your horse's behaviour, as these could be indications of underlying emotional issues. Neglecting such issues could lead to physical health problems. It is, therefore, imperative to be mindful of your horse's emotional state and take appropriate measures to address any concerns. Here are some specific points to consider when monitoring its emotional wellbeing.

EXERCISE
The horse's exercise and competition schedule should not push them to their limits. They require adequate rest for both their body and mind. Allowing at least two full days of rest per week is

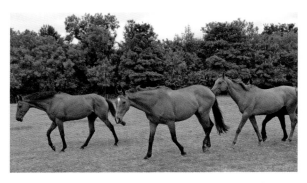

Socialising and interacting in a herd is critical for horses to express their innate behaviours, have enjoyable experiences, take breaks and engage in natural exercise with their peers. These activities play a vital role in their emotional well-being, as evidenced by my two horses, Joe and Shamus, who are leading the herd.

essential for every horse and, after intensive work, a recovery period of forty-eight hours should be observed to facilitate muscle recuperation. It is often underestimated how demanding it is for a horse to learn new movements, maintain a competition frame, travel and compete. Many of these horses experience mental and physical fatigue and may also carry underlying discomfort.

WEANING AND BACKING
I frequently encounter horses which, at approximately six years of age, begin to lose interest in their work and exhibit challenging behaviour. This behaviour can stem from physical discomfort or emotional disturbances caused by inadequate weaning and harsh or premature backing. Horses that have experienced a disrespectful start in life may display aggressive behaviour and emotional issues that can have long-term consequences. It is crucial to establish a solid foundation for young horses through proper weaning, backing and training. When considering the purchase of a horse, it is essential to gather information about its early history to mitigate potential problems.

Lastly, when horses exhibit more severe behaviours such as complete shutdown, biting, barging or rearing, they are expressing their distress as

I once treated a mare that suffered from severe back pain and developed a fear of the saddle due to a cruel weaning and backing process during her time with a dealer. Consequently, she could not be ridden and had to live solely as a brood mare. In such cases, it is crucial to provide the horse with manual therapy and establish bonding exercises to cultivate trust and happiness. If re-backing is a viable option, it may require significant time and perseverance, but the process is worthwhile when approached with empathy. However, I strongly advise against entrusting this task to others unless they come highly recommended and you can closely monitor the process. I have witnessed numerous beautiful horses given a second chance to live happily with the right owner. Regrettably, I have also encountered instances in which horses were unjustly deemed dangerous due to their challenging beginnings, leading to their euthanasia instead of receiving the kindness and love they truly needed.

loudly as possible, desperately seeking attention. Ignoring their signals only exacerbates the behaviour and worsens the situation.

TRANSITING YARDS

Frequent relocation can stress horses, causing anxiety, fear and depression. It can also expose them to new diseases and parasites, increasing the risk of illness. Consider your horse's physical and emotional wellbeing before relocating it. Ensure the new yard provides adequate care, nutrition and socialisation. I once worked with an eventing horse that showed signs of depression due to constant relocation. It caused him to frequently lose his companions and security, affecting his wellbeing and performance. After his final relocation, he was so traumatised that

he never returned to eventing.

The frequent relocation of horses between yards can lead to emotional turmoil, particularly when they have formed friendships and established a place within the herd. Owners must reflect on the reasons for moving their horses; if the decision solely serves their interest and does not entirely benefit the horse, they should reconsider.

PEER INFLUENCE

All horses should be treated as individuals according to their needs, which vary from horse to horse. No horse owner should feel peer influence or pressure to treat their horses in a particular way. If a horse owner is a novice, getting professional help and accessing as much education as possible is better than relying on others who give well meaning but often conflicting or inaccurate advice.

Regrettably, I have observed instances where a cob, for example, was trained in the same manner as a thoroughbred due to peer pressure, which is not acceptable as they are different breeds and possess distinct anatomical characteristics necessitating different types of exercise to avoid pain and injury.

ANTHROPOMORPHISM

Anthropomorphism is the act of ascribing human qualities, emotions and goals to non-humans. Some people see themselves as their horse, with human needs, ideas and feelings, instead of the horse's unique species. Examples of horse anthropomorphism include:

'My horse is jealous because he saw me riding my friend's horse yesterday' – we have no scientific evidence that horses display jealousy this way.

'My horse rears just to get me off' – usually, a horse rears only when they are in discomfort, and you need to find out why.

Horses experience a range of human emotions, including grief, fear, pain, frustration, anger, anxiety, depression, sadness, loneliness, happiness, excitement, contentment and playfulness, but differences in brain function prevent us from processing information similarly. When a horse exhibits unwanted behaviour, it is important for the owner to step back and determine why. The most natural, positive or progressive-minded horse people tend not to anthropomorphise whilst understanding that their horse does feel emotions. The more you learn to 'read' your horse, the better your partnership.

BREED AND CONFORMATION

Another factor influencing management is the horse's breed and conformation traits and whether they are fit for purpose for the equestrian discipline intended for it. If not, the horse will succumb to performance failure and eventually pain and injury. Having the correct conformation will improve the horse's performance, reduce the risk of injury, improve athletic ability, control and manoeuvrability, and increase comfort for both the horse and the rider.

RE-TRAINING FOR ANOTHER DISCIPLINE

Thoroughbreds are versatile for other equestrian disciplines, and we see many racehorse-to-riding horse successes, but the transition needs to be done correctly. It should be planned with flexibility in case setbacks occur and a timescale based on the horse's individual needs.

There is no quick fix when retraining a racehorse. The six- to eight-week turnaround time seen often in the industry by those wanting to make quick money needs to be reviewed. I would never recommend buying a horse from a dealer or anyone who has rushed this transition. I have found horses that have initially been rushed during retraining and passed on to an owner too quickly, often resulting in problems in the future. It is never the horse's fault but those doing the retraining incorrectly. Some former racehorses take months or years to retrain. It is certainly not for a novice or anyone wanting a quick profit.

All former racehorses need a period of relaxation and turnout to allow the demands of racing and its rigid regime to leave them before embarking on a retraining programme. During the retraining, the horse will use different muscles than when racing. Many muscles will have been overtrained, and others will be undertrained. This can cause immense tension for the horse during this emotionally and physically demanding period of change if it is not done carefully and considerately.

I have been involved with many former racehorses embarking on a new discipline. They all need support as they often carry injuries from racing, some minor and some major, which might be known to the new owner or might not be apparent until the retraining process begins, when they expect the horse to be able to do things that it cannot. Osteoarthritis, tendon injuries, trigger points in muscles, muscle tears and scar tissue are often evident in former racehorses due to the demands of their discipline. However, this can be managed and, in many instances, does not prevent the horse from excelling in a new life. Manual therapy and correct supportive exercise are essential for racehorses retraining for another discipline.

I recall a woman who bought a racehorse from the horse sales and paid £400; she brought him home to retrain; her plan was to train him for six weeks and then sell him on and make a profit and get another one. Sadly, I have seen this so many times.

The horse started to rear as she attempted to ride him in a collected frame, a week after its last race, yet he would have no idea how to 'collect', as this was a long way off. The woman contacted me to check him over because she said he was being 'naughty'.

I found the horse to have emotional and physical tension in its muscles but a fantastic personality, as so many horses possess. I explained to the woman that there was no place for a quick fix with horses, and he needed time. I checked the saddle, and it was pinching the horse; she had used one that belonged to another of her horses. I suggested she give the horse a month of turnout, then start it slowly but not to ride the horse until its back recovered – and certainly not in that saddle.

A week later, I was informed by another person at the yard that she had ridden the horse in the saddle that did not fit, he had reared, and she had fallen off. She beat the horse and sold him to the abattoir 'meat man'. I was disgusted, and I certainly let my feelings be known.

It is unfortunate when a good horse goes to waste due to a lack of proper management, patience and knowledge. With the right approach, such horses could have become wonderful partners. However, many horses are subjected to quick retraining and sold for a profit, often resulting in their potential being unfulfilled. It is crucial to recognise the importance of time, patience and knowledge in developing a horse's full potential. By refusing to buy horses subjected to such practices, we can reduce the demand and encourage a more responsible and ethical approach to horse training and ownership. Ultimately, this will benefit the horses, the industry, and the equestrian community.

What Happens When the Horse's Natural Needs Are Not Met?

When basic management or natural needs are not met, it can lead to various negative consequences. The horse's physical health is compromised, and behaviour problems arise as 'vices' or stereotypies, anxiety and possibly aggression. Their performance decreases, as does their lifespan.

UNWANTED BEHAVIOURS (STEREOTYPIES)

Stereotypies are repetitive behaviours observed in domesticated horses resulting from unpleasant stimuli such as fear or pain. They are not seen in their wild counterparts. Examples include crib-biting, wind-sucking, weaving, box-walking, and self-mutilation. Owners should work to eliminate the cause of the behaviour rather than resort to devices such as windsucking collars. Manual therapy helps with both the physical and emotional effects of stereotypies. For instance, windsucking and crib-biting can cause inflammation in the neck muscles and throat, leading to breathing difficulties and muscular issues when ridden in flexion. Weaving and box-walking can cause tension in the neck and shoulder muscles and even osteoarthritis in the knees. Box-walking in a circular motion can cause asymmetry and unbalanced muscle build-up. Studies have shown that cortisol levels can rise significantly when a horse moves like this in a circle.

Addressing physical or behavioural issues as soon as they arise helps prevent problems from escalating and becoming more difficult to solve. Early intervention also ensures the horse's wellbeing and can improve the human–horse relationship. Additionally, it can prevent health issues, such as lameness, from developing into chronic conditions and decreasing performance. A well-rounded management programme with manual therapy and bespoke training that considers the horse's needs and abilities can help maintain and improve performance.

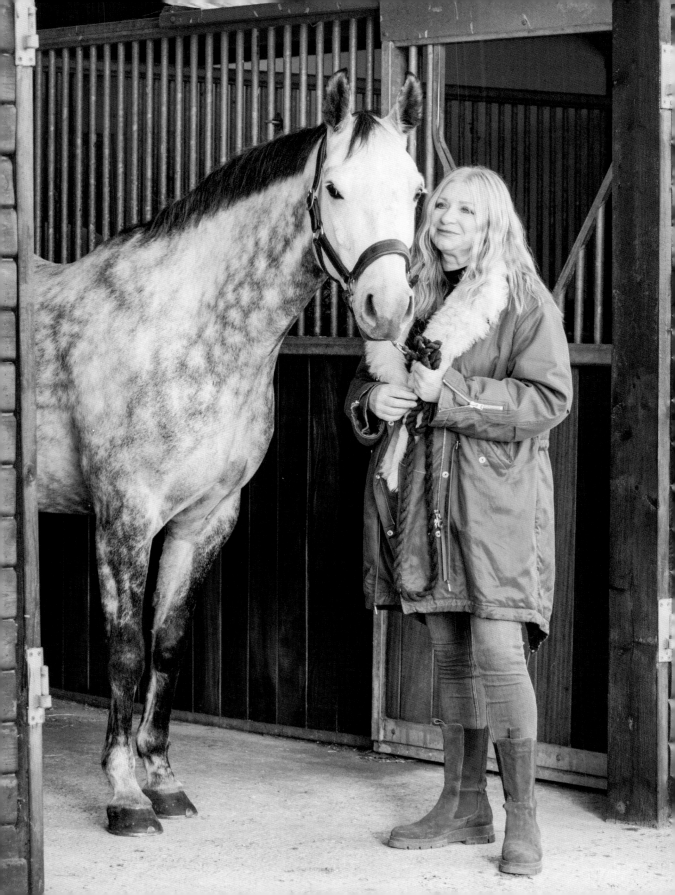

CHAPTER 2

The Benefits of
Musculoskeletal 'Manual' Therapy

The terms musculoskeletal therapist, manual therapist, bodyworker, physiotherapist and massage therapist can refer to the professionals who offer this therapy to horses. While they provide similar therapy, their methods and skill sets may differ depending on their level of training. When horse owners administer therapy to their horses, I typically refer to it as manual therapy.

Musculoskeletal therapists address the relationship between muscles, fascia, connective tissue, joints and bones and how these elements work in conjunction to maintain the horse's health and athletic ability. The fundamental principle is that if any of these components are impaired due to overuse, tension, inflexibility, immune deficiency or toxicity, the entire musculoskeletal system is adversely affected.

Expert therapists can also provide targeted exercises that prioritise biomechanical and structural training or rehabilitation of the horse, which is covered in Chapter 8. This targeted approach optimises the horse's functional movement, allowing it to excel in its career and cope with any earlier improper training, conformation weaknesses, and other conditions that can result in chronic injury or degeneration. Furthermore, this specialised therapy has a positive impact on the emotional and physical wellbeing of the horse, rendering it invaluable for its wellbeing.

This chapter will cover the primary factors that necessitate a horse needing therapy and the advantages it provides to the entire horse.

Benefits to the Horse as an Athlete

An equine athlete is characterised by their proficiency and skill in the exercises and unique demands of a particular equestrian discipline or sport, which necessitates strength, agility and stamina. To excel in any undertaking, a horse must have unrestricted mobility, flexibility and be free from discomfort. Even if a horse does not compete, it can still be regarded as an athlete by executing manoeuvres while bearing the weight of a rider, which is a remarkable athletic achievement.

The competitive demand for horses appears to be increasing rapidly. Unfortunately, this also means that horses are subjected to considerable loading and stress, which can compromise their musculoskeletal system. For most horse owners, the prospect of their horse getting injured is their worst nightmare. Injuries not only cause pain to the horse but also delay training and competition schedules, can be expensive to treat, and in the long run, can lead to a decrease in performance and the likelihood of further injury.

While damaged tissues may eventually heal, they can take a toll on the horse's body. When muscles are pushed to their limits through athletic tasks, the chances of re-injury and the development of permanent conditions increase. Furthermore, dealing with injuries can be extremely frustrating and exhausting for owners, especially if they require ongoing management.

Benefits to Body Systems

For competitive equestrians, implementing a comprehensive horse care plan that includes regular manual therapy can provide a competitive edge and reduce the risk of injuries. Even recreational horses can benefit from regular manual therapy, which can increase their flexibility and overall health, leading to a longer and healthier life with fewer ailments. For these reasons, we highly recommend that horse owners incorporate manual therapy into their horse's health care regime. By doing so, they can implement a preventative injury protocol, minimising the risk of injuries and the subsequent negative impact on the horse's performance and wellbeing.

As noted in Chapter 1, the various body systems of horses are interconnected, and manual therapy can have a positive impact on all of them. Looking at some systems specifically:

THE MUSCULOSKELETAL SYSTEM

Manual therapy has numerous benefits for a horse's musculoskeletal system. It can help to reduce muscle tension and stiffness, which can lead to improved flexibility, range of motion and comfort. Additionally, it can improve muscle tone and condition, promoting overall muscular health and function. Moreover, it can be an effective tool for supporting the healing process after an injury or surgery, promoting increased circulation and nutrient supply and reducing inflammation and waste product accumulation. Many horses have undiagnosed peripheral nerve lesions; these can be assisted by encouraging blood flow to denervated tissues.

Manual therapy can be particularly advantageous for horses involved in high-intensity athletic activi-

ties, as it aids in enhancing performance. Addressing compensatory changes, it assists in rebalancing the horse's muscle groups, improving posture, increasing overall flexibility and reducing muscle pain. Notably, a 2010 study demonstrated that manual therapy applied to the muscles of the hindquarters resulted in a significant increase in stride length. Subsequent research has made significant progress, providing more positive findings to support the efficacy of manual therapy for horses.

Lastly, manual therapy effectively reduces muscle tension by promoting an increased parasympathetic response in horses. This relaxation is often evidenced by horses closing their eyes, dropping their lip and exhibiting slow and steady breathing.

THE NERVOUS SYSTEM

The horse's nervous system is a complex network of nerves and cells composed of two main parts, the central nervous system (CNS) and the peripheral nervous system (PNS). The central nervous system includes the brain and the spinal cord, which are responsible for processing and coordinating sensory information and sending motor commands to various parts of the body. It is the control centre of the entire nervous system. The PNS consists of the nerves that connect the CNS to the rest of the body. It is further divided into two branches: the somatic nervous system and the autonomic nervous system. The somatic nervous system is responsible for voluntary movements and sensations, such as the horse's ability to move its legs or feel the touch of a rider's leg. The autonomic nervous system controls involuntary functions, such as heart rate, breathing and digestion. It is further divided into the sympathetic and parasympathetic branches, which have opposing effects on the body. The sympathetic branch is responsible for the 'fight or flight' response, while the parasympathetic is responsible for the 'rest and digest' response.

Manual therapy can have a number of benefits and positive effects on the body's nervous system. Firstly, a generalised relaxation response occurs that helps

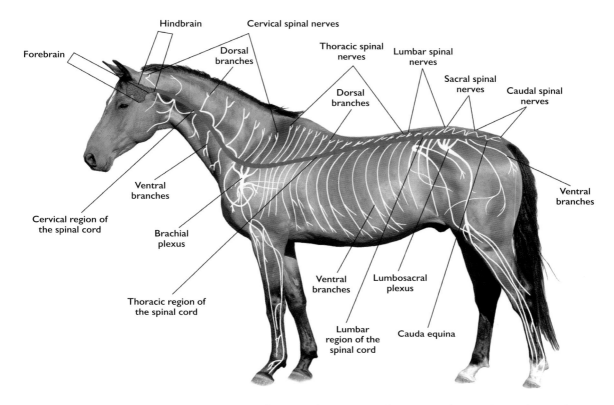

The horse's nervous system, whereby the CNS and PNS work together to regulate and coordinate the horse's movements and bodily functions. Nerves can become impinged due to various factors, such as incorrect saddle fit or injuries resulting in compression or irritation of the nerves.

reduce strain on the nervous system. Secondly, it can help in the reduction of pain due to stimulating the release of endorphins. Thirdly, it can help to reduce fascial and muscular tension as well as the reduction of joint stiffness, which can release impingement of peripheral nerves. Finally, manual therapy can help reduce the horse's time in 'sympathetic overdrive' or 'fight or flight'.

THE CIRCULATORY SYSTEM

The circulatory system of a horse is responsible for the transportation of oxygen, nutrients and hormones throughout its body. It comprises the heart, blood vessels and blood, and serves as the horse's internal transportation network. The heart pumps oxygen-depleted blood to the lungs, where it is oxygenated and returned to the heart; the heart then pumps oxygen-rich blood throughout the body, delivering nutrients and oxygen to the horse's cells and removing waste products. The circulatory system also plays a crucial role in regulating the horse's body temperature, pH balance, and immune system.

Manual therapy can have several benefits for a horse's circulatory system. Firstly, it can help to increase blood flow and oxygenation to the muscles, which can improve their overall health and performance. This increased blood flow can also aid in the removal of waste products and toxins from the muscles, further promoting their health. It can also help to reduce muscle tension and stiffness, which can improve the elasticity of blood vessels and increase their ability to dilate. This can lead to better circulation and nutrient delivery throughout the body.

The exact number of blood vessels – arteries, veins and capillaries – varies depending on the size and weight of the horse. On average a horse's circulatory system can contain approximately 60,000 to 80,000 miles of blood vessels. This extensive network allows for the exchange of oxygen, nutrients and waste products between the blood and the tissues in the horse's body.

Another essential part of the circulatory system is the lymphatic system, responsible for immune function and waste removal. It is a network of vessels and organs that help to transport lymph, a clear fluid that contains lymphocytes and other immune cells throughout the body. Lymphocytes can be found within the lymph nodes, which are small, bean-shaped structures that act as filters, trapping and removing harmful substances such as bacteria and viruses from the lymphatic fluid. They play a crucial role in the immune response.

Manual therapy can stimulate and improve lymphatic flow, whereby inflammation and swelling in the body are reduced, supporting the overall health of the circulatory system. It can also help release restrictions on circulatory flow, reduce oedema and bruising, and induce the parasympathetic response, which slows and strengthens the heartbeat, promoting the 'rest and digest' activity.

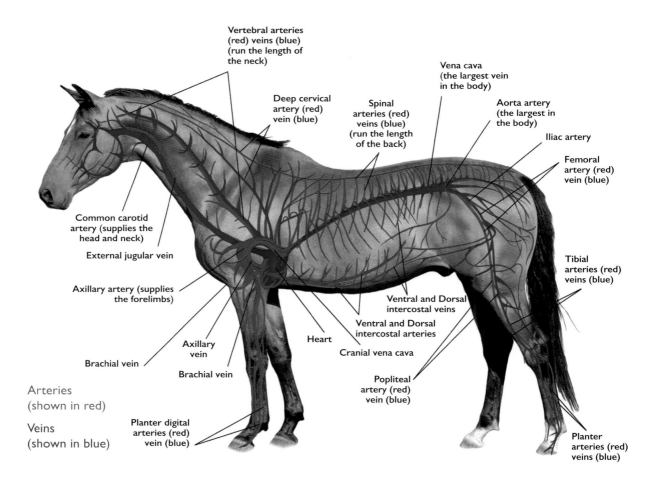

Veins carry blood back to the heart, while arteries carry blood away from the heart. The length and complexity of the circulatory system reflect the high demands placed on a powerful animal, which needs a robust blood supply to fuel its muscles and organs during exercise and other activities.

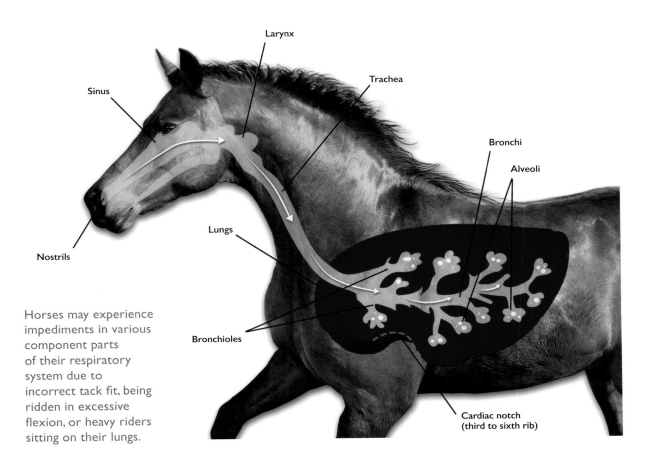

Larynx

Trachea

Sinus

Bronchi

Alveoli

Nostrils

Lungs

Bronchioles

Cardiac notch
(third to sixth rib)

Horses may experience impediments in various component parts of their respiratory system due to incorrect tack fit, being ridden in excessive flexion, or heavy riders sitting on their lungs.

THE RESPIRATORY SYSTEM

The horse's respiratory system is a biological system consisting of a series of organs responsible for taking in oxygen and expelling carbon dioxide. The primary organs of the respiratory system are the lungs, which carry out this exchange of gases as the horse breathes. When the horse breathes, its lungs filter in the oxygen and pass it through the bloodstream, which carries it into the tissues and organs. Lungs also remove carbon dioxide from the blood, releasing it into the air when breathing out.

Manual therapy can have several benefits on the horse's respiratory system. It can relax the tension in the diaphragm and encourage deeper breathing, which improves diaphragm function. It can also lessen hypertonicity, which is severe tension in the intercostal muscles and muscles in the chest, back and neck areas, thus increasing rib cage mobility and the metabolism in the lungs. Finally, by inducing the parasympathetic response, it produces deeper and more efficient breathing. This response can also decrease the symptoms of some respiratory tract diseases, such as equine asthma.

THE DIGESTIVE SYSTEM

The horse's digestive system involves a complex process that relies upon the breakdown of food in several stages. The horse chews its food and mixes it with saliva to create a bolus that is then swallowed. The food then passes through the oesophagus and into the stomach, where it is mixed with stomach acid and enzymes. From there, the partially digested food moves into the small intestine, where most of the nutrient absorption occurs. The food then enters the large intestine, which is made up of the caecum, colon and rectum. The caecum is the largest part of the large intestine and plays a crucial role in the digestion of

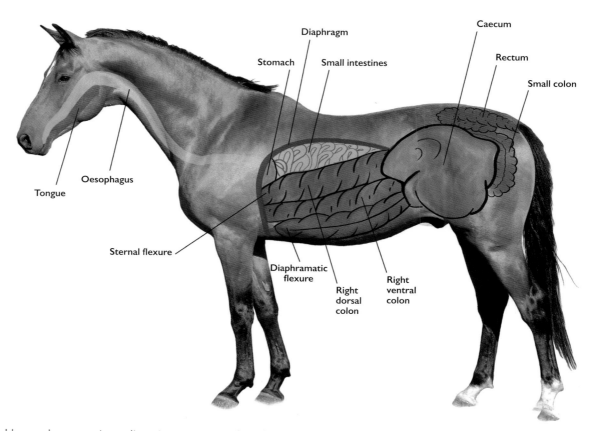

Diaphragm
Caecum
Stomach
Small intestines
Rectum
Small colon
Oesophagus
Tongue
Sternal flexure
Diaphramatic flexure
Right dorsal colon
Right ventral colon

Horses have a unique digestive system in that they are 'hindgut fermenters', which means that most of their digestion takes place in the large intestine rather than the stomach. This makes them particularly sensitive to changes in their diet.

plant material through the fermentation of cellulose by symbiotic microorganisms. The colon is responsible for the absorption of water and electrolytes and the formation and storage of faeces. The rectum is the final part of the large intestine, where faeces are eliminated through the rectum.

Manual therapy can help the horse's digestive system by promoting relaxation, reducing tension and increasing blood flow to the gastrointestinal tract. This can stimulate the digestive system, enhance nutrient absorption and alleviate symptoms of gastrointestinal disorders such as constipation and impaction colic.

THE SKIN AND COAT

Manual therapy increases blood flow by bringing fresh oxygen and nutrients to the skin. This also encourages the presence of healing red blood cells nourishing and brightening the coat and decreasing inflammation. Therefore, manual therapy can be more beneficial than chemical products to help a horse's coat appear glossier.

Benefits with Conformation Deviations

Examining a horse's conformation is important as it relates to its biomechanics and performance. Conformation refers to a horse's physical structure and proportions, which varies greatly within and between different breeds. While perfect conformation does not guarantee performance or soundness, it can assist in predicting possible musculoskeletal strengths and weaknesses and predisposition to injury or musculoskeletal disorders.

Many horses suffer from orthopaedic health issues due to conformation weaknesses and equestrian demands. Good conformation affects the potential for biomechanical efficiency, better performance and musculoskeletal durability, so it is important to look for horses with specific conformation traits when competing at elite levels. If a horse lacks ideal conformation, careful management can prevent joint wear and tear, promoting soundness.

Biomechanics studies the mechanical aspects of biological systems, including how muscles, fascia, bones, tendons and ligaments work together to produce movement. Many books are written on the subject, and it is not my intention to delve too deeply here into equine biomechanics, except for its relationship with conformation, performance and manual therapy.

Here are some ways that I have seen a horse's conformation affect its biomechanics and performance:

Movement – including its gait and stride length. For example, horses with longer legs and a more sloping shoulder may be able to cover more ground with each stride, while horses with a shorter stride may have to work harder to maintain the same speed.

Balance and coordination – horses with a well-balanced conformation may be more agile and able to perform complex manoeuvres, while horses with a less-balanced conformation may struggle with balance and coordination.

Flexibility and range of motion – for example, horses with a more upright pastern and steeper shoulder may have less range of motion in their front legs, while horses with a more sloping shoulder and longer pasterns may have more range of motion.

Weight distribution – horses with a heavier front end may struggle with collection and balance, while horses with a heavier hind end may have more power and drive from behind.

Injury risk – this can be higher. For example, horses with a long back may be more prone to back pain; an upright shoulder might limit stride length and place strain on the front limbs; over at the knee can cause stress to the front limbs and increase the risk of tendonitis and ligament injuries; weak pasterns might cause chronic lameness and suspensory ligament injuries; and cow hocks can cause a higher risk of strain on the hock joints.

Thus, it is crucial for horse owners to understand their horse's conformation, its strengths and weaknesses and develop a tailored management and training plan that considers these factors, including appropriate exercise and manual therapy. Regrettably, many horses are labelled 'loss of use' or euthanised due to preventable injuries caused by poor management.

I have seen many horses with a conformation deviation in the lower limb, such as toe-in (pigeon toe), which has put pressure on joints over time and has caused biomechanical or gait alternations such as paddling (outward swinging of the foot). This conformation and biomechanical action has further resulted in crooked bones in the lower limb, eventually leading to conditions such as bone fractures or degeneration, as in osteoarthritis. These horses have been able to cope with low-level work but not heavier work. By providing regular manual therapy and adjusting the workload, I have managed to keep them as sound as possible, and this is how owners can help their horses to live a more comfortable and lengthy existence.

Comparing Desirable and Undesirable Conformations

When buying horses or breeding from them, we should consider any inherited conformational negatives or weaknesses and whether they will potentially hinder performance and require specific management. The most heritable conformation traits that need specific management that I have seen in my career are poor foot conformations, over at the knee or back at the knee, toe in or toe out, upright pasterns or sloping pasterns, sickle hocks or straight hocks.

There are many books written on conformation and how to assess it, and it is not my intention to provide a detailed analysis of conformation; instead, the point is to emphasise that a horse, as an athlete, needs regular manual therapy, especially if it is challenged with conformation traits that cause weakness. Also, an owner must consider their expectations of the horse and what the horse must do mechanically to meet them. Will its conformation inhibit or support such athletic abilities?

There are many methods of assessing conformation for the ideals, from a simple plumb line system to complex geometry. As a good basis, horses should be as symmetrical as possible, in balance, with a good size and length of the bone. To a degree, minor conformation flaws are manageable if the horse is not overworked, but significant flaws can be more challenging at any functional level.

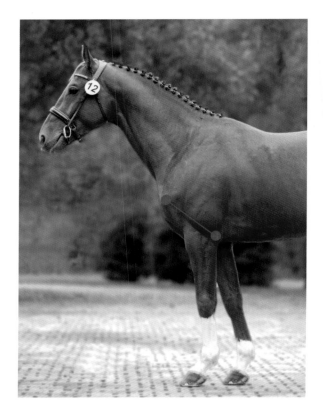

This chestnut horse has an angled humerus, shown by the red line, which indicates that the point of the shoulder is much higher than the elbow; the steep angle means it can fold its knees up quickly and high. This will enhance its jumping ability.

SHOULDER CONFORMATION FOR JUMPING HORSES

When a horse is required to jump in its equestrian discipline, it needs to rotate its scapula to lift the point of shoulder, move the elbow forward and lift its knees over a fence. Depending on the angle of the point of shoulder and elbow, as indicated in the images with the red dots, the horse's front legs will react differently.

LUMBOSACRAL JOINT (LSJ) STRENGTHS AND WEAKNESSES

Anatomically, the lumbosacral junction is the area where the horse's back and hindquarters meet. It is characterised by the forward-facing spinous processes in the lumbar vertebrae, while those in the sacral ver-

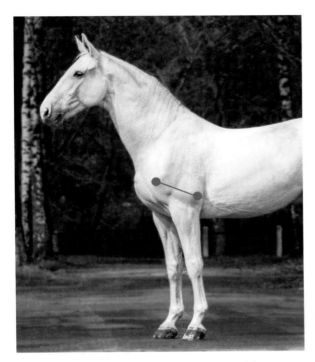

This grey horse has a lower point of shoulder; as such, its forehand will be slower to lift the knees over a fence, with less height than that of the chestnut horse. This will hinder its jumping ability.

When considering the conformation of the lumbosacral joint (LSJ), the palpable areas are the tuber sacrale (croup) and the tuber coxae (the point of hip); it is the angle between the two that is important. A well-placed LSJ can be an asset to a horse in terms of its athleticism and ability to engage its hindquarters and transfer all its power from its hindquarters forward and upward.

Injuries in the lumbosacral junction (LSJ) are common in all horses, especially those involved in performance disciplines. If left untreated, these injuries can lead to long-term bone degeneration, another reason to address problems in this area promptly. Several causes contribute to LSJ issues, primarily stemming from inadequate man-

tebrae face toward the tail. This arrangement creates a distinct 'V' shape, known as the lumbosacral junction. This junction plays a crucial role as it allows the horse to bring its hind legs under its body, serving as a transmission point for forward motion and compensating for other weaknesses.

It is considered one of the most important aspects of functional conformation, as it enables flexion (rounding) and extension (hollowing) of the horse's back, compensating for the limited range of motion in the backbones. An 'upwardly flexed topline' is when the abdominal muscles contract and lift the back. This position is less strenuous on the horse's body when it is ridden. Conversely, an undesirable posture known as a 'downwardly flexed topline' or hollow, weakens the horse's back and makes it difficult to support a rider. This position is more taxing on the horse's structure and brings the vertebrae closer together. Chapter 4 gives examples of such ridden frames.

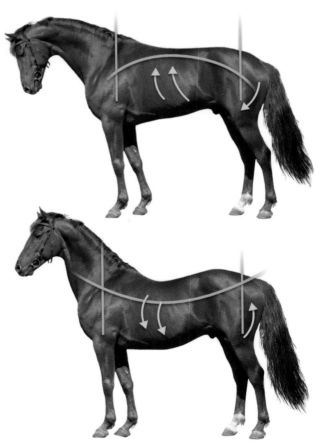

The top image illustrates the ideal posture for a horse, referred to as an 'upwardly flexed topline'; the bottom image shows a 'downwardly flexed topline'.

agement practices such as incorrectly fitting saddles, over-training, injuries or falls, and rushing the horse back into work too quickly. Improper riding techniques and a lack of regular checks and musculoskeletal therapy by a qualified professional can also contribute to LSJ problems. Horses with less-than-ideal conformation of the LSJ for their respective disciplines are more likely to experience frequent issues. While well-trained musculoskeletal therapists can provide assistance, there are cases where veterinary intervention becomes necessary.

In the following images, the anatomical landmark of the LSJ is indicated by a yellow dot and the tuber coxae with a white dot.

I have seen horses that are built to perform a specific job tend to learn it more efficiently and display fewer resistances to their training. As a result, they are less prone to performance-related injuries. This is not restricted to those performing at elite levels: it also applies to recreational horses who do little more than a hack; both tend to have longer careers, be it a competitive one or through advancing years.

Those that require specific management due to their less-than-ideal conformations require constant monitoring, musculoskeletal therapy provided by a professional and regular review of the type and duration of exercise to avoid repetitive strain injury and deterioration of already vulnerable body parts.

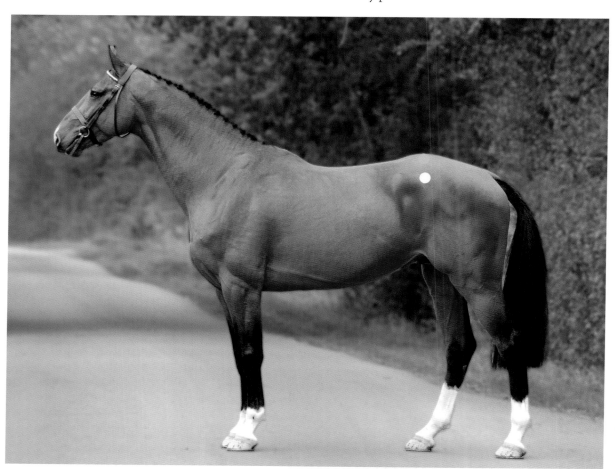

LSJ positioned above the tuber coxae provides for maximum athleticism and power. This could be considered the ideal position.

MUSCLE HEALTH AND BIOMECHANICS

Muscles serve to propel the horse and stabilise it. For every muscle that moves a joint in one direction, a counter muscle can pull the joint in the other direction. When the opposing muscles work in unison, both activating in balance, they stabilise joints. This keeps the legs rigid when weight bearing, the back from breaking, and the head elevated and in motion with the horse's movement.

Using electromyography, research reveals that muscles, during the walk, trot and canter, must work in equilibrium to create movement. If one muscle is tight, injured or restricted, this could affect balance and movement. Also, subtle lameness in the horse's fore-limbs and hindlimbs causes changes in the pelvis and back during movement. If the muscles are not working in equilibrium, it will have a compensatory effect on the horse's musculoskeletal system, affecting gait patterns.

Before an owner can undertake an accurate assessment of how their horse is moving and whether this might be caused by a conformation weakness, is biomechanical or a combination of both, which is commonly the case, they must know exactly what constitutes good biomechanics of gait to compare when there could be an abnormality.

Unless you have access to gait analysis equipment used in several studies, the best way to assess gait is to video the horse in slow motion and critique it afterwards. Unfortunately, the naked eye will not see in real time what a slow-motion video will.

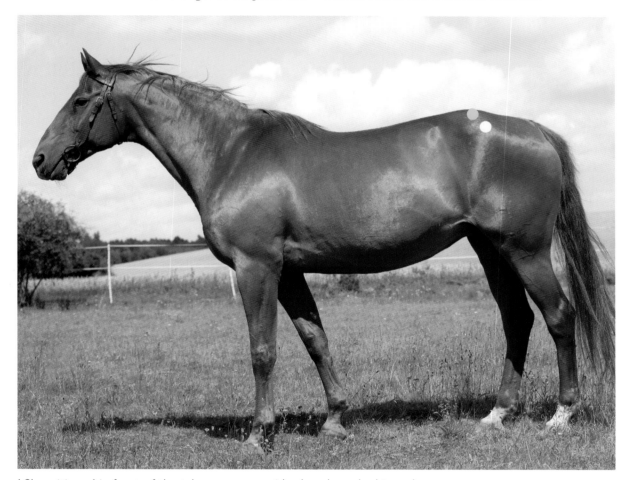

LSJ positioned in front of the tuber coxae provides length to the hip and power potential and is suitable for engagement of the hindquarters.

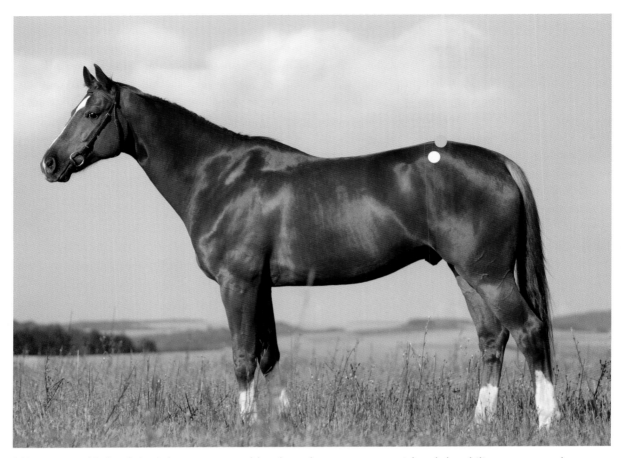

LSJ positioned behind the tuber coxae would reduce the power potential and the ability to engage the hindquarters. Horses in this category are often prone to back problems.

When I have been presented with a musculoskeletal problem, and I link this to how the horse moves, many horse owners say, 'The horse has always moved like that' or 'That's the way he is.' This may be true, but it does not mean it is correct, and more often than not, the horse is displaying a biomechanical deficit, putting it at risk of injury and degeneration. If any horse does not move correctly, there will be a cause and an effect highly likely to result in pain. Any abnormalities in gait should be addressed and helped by manual therapy and other interventions if required. When assessing potential problems, the following gaits are the most reliable.

The Walk

In the walk, the horse moves its head up and down to help maintain its balance by working like a pendulum.

It is, therefore, essential not to restrict the horse's head; otherwise, this affects its balance. If the head is restricted, it will use other body parts to help balance, which is where problems in its musculoskeletal system can begin. We accept that many disciplines require the horse to have its head held in flexion, but that does not mean it is correct. It is for such reasons that I do not condone horses being held in for long periods or tied in with training aids in ridden and lunging work, as it only causes problems in the long term.

When the walk is abnormal, we know the horse is uncomfortable and unable to maintain a correct walk. The horse will reduce the load on the problem limb and nod or raise its head accordingly and might hold its tail crooked, also indicating the use of its tail for balance and pain being present.

The Trot

When the trot is abnormal, there is an irregularity of the rhythm; the horse might be stepping short and not tracking up, look crooked, hold its head higher with a hollow back, it might nod, drag its limbs, and its tail might be held to one side. This motion would be uncomfortable for the horse, the vertebrae would be closer together when the head is raised, and the back is hollow, which reduces strength and movement in the entire back region and negatively affects the pelvis and the neck. This is another example of how very quickly horses can be in pain and break down if their gait is abnormal.

The Canter

When the canter is abnormal, the moment of suspension appears briefly or is missing, and the gait becomes four-beat. The horse might fall in when cantering on a circle, look crooked when cantering, canter on the wrong lead, look disunited behind, and possibly drag limbs. The horse's head should never have a very high head carriage with a dipped back in canter. Canter is the best gait to assess a horse for sacroiliac problems, often identified as a 'bunny hopping' gait in which the hind legs move together; this can be better seen on the lunge.

Jumping

When the horse has insufficient impulsion and poor balance, it can land heavily on its front legs, making it challenging to resume the canter, and on a deep or slippery surface, it can lead to the horse falling. If the horse jumps with a stiff, hollow back or retracted neck, this prevents a good bascule and causes a stiff, inhibited jump. Without a good bascule, the forelegs cannot be lifted as high or folded as tightly and also, the hind legs may trail too low, which means they often hit the fence. In addition, some horses land unevenly because one of their limbs is sore. A horse might also refuse to jump because it anticipates pain.

Moving on a Circle (on a lunge)

This is another good way to assess a horse but it is not my preferred exercise method. If a horse is to be lunged for exercise purposes, then the entire surface of the school should be used. Horses do not move well in a circle; their anatomy is not designed for it, which is why I am not a fan of circular horse-walkers – I prefer the oblong or oval design.

When moving correctly on a circle, the inside front and hind leg make a smaller circle than the outside front, and hind leg and the horse should have a good bend through the neck, back and hindquarters following the shape of the circle. The head and neck should appear relaxed, and the horse should step under with the inside hind leg and have a correct rhythm for the moving gait. The horse should move equally on both reins. If not, there is potential for problems.

When a horse moves abnormally on the inside of a circle, any lameness in a leg becomes more apparent. This is because the horse tends to shift more weight onto the inside leg, which accentuates the lameness. As a result, the horse's movement on one rein may appear shorter compared to the other. In addition, there may be issues with overbending or insufficient bending through the neck, back and hindquarters.

If your horse displays abnormal gaits or movements, then reassess using slow-motion video, and on a different surface; you should compare moving on a softer surface with a firmer surface. If the horse displays an abnormal gait on a softer surface, it is usually associated with its upper body, muscles and soft tissues. If it shows an abnormal movement on a firmer surface, it is usually bone related, often in the limbs. Whether the problem originates in the soft tissues or bone, the horse will compensate in its movement, protecting itself from pain.

After assessing the gait, thoroughly palpate the horse to find areas of muscle tension; this is a good test to compare with what you see and feel. Then provide your manual therapy accordingly and regularly to maintain the horse. If you suspect degeneration, such as osteoarthritis, you might want to investigate further through veterinary diagnostics.

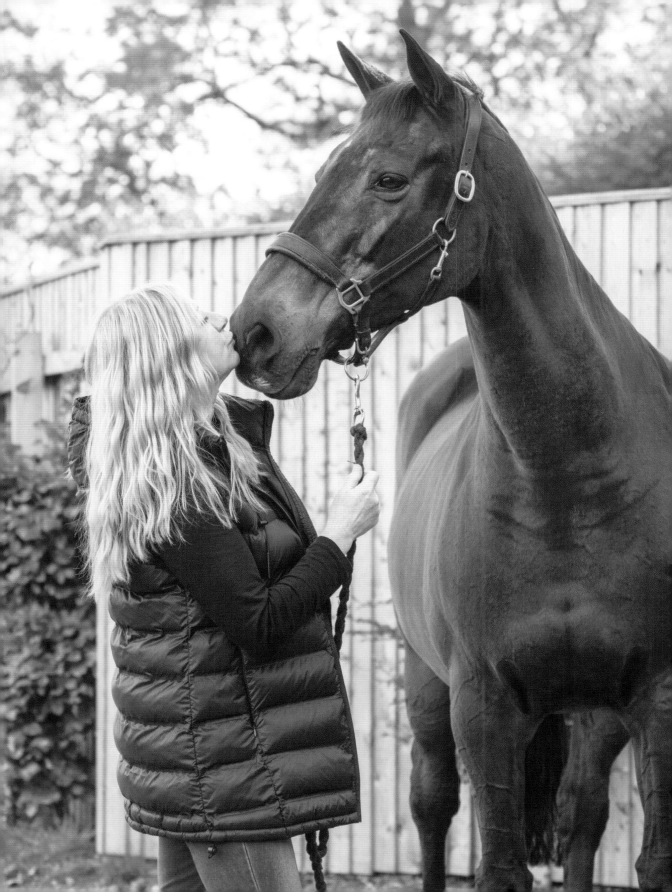

CHAPTER 3

Equine Anatomy

Equine anatomy refers to the physical structure and organisation of the horse's body, and having a basic understanding of anatomy is essential for horse owners to provide the best care they can for their horses and for those who will be following my guidance in this book by undertaking manual therapy on them. This chapter will focus specifically on the skeletal and muscular systems, due to their relevance in manual therapy work and the correct training of horses.

The Skeletal System

The horse's skeleton has many positive features, such as its ability to support the animal's weight and provide a strong framework for muscle attachment, enabling the horse to move and perform various activities. Additionally, the horse's bones are adapted to withstand significant forces and stresses.

The horse's skeleton also has negative aspects.

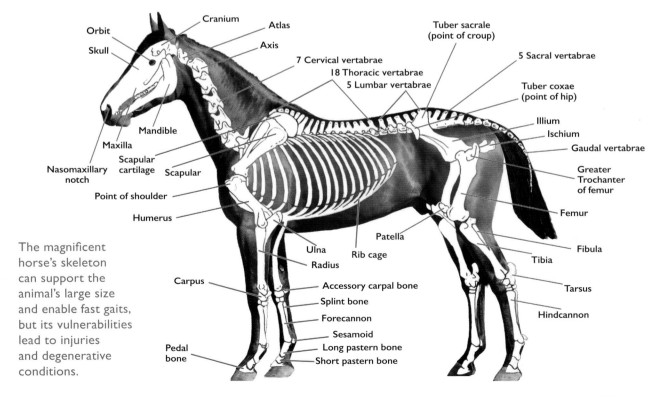

The magnificent horse's skeleton can support the animal's large size and enable fast gaits, but its vulnerabilities lead to injuries and degenerative conditions.

Cranium
Orbit
Atlas
Skull
Axis
7 Cervical vertabrae
18 Thoracic vertabrae
5 Lumbar vertabrae
Tuber sacrale (point of croup)
5 Sacral vertabrae
Tuber coxae (point of hip)
Illium
Ischium
Gaudal vertabrae
Greater Trochanter of femur
Femur
Fibula
Tibia
Tarsus
Hindcannon
Patella
Mandible
Maxilla
Scapular cartilage
Scapular
Nasomaxillary notch
Point of shoulder
Humerus
Ulna
Rib cage
Radius
Carpus
Accessory carpal bone
Splint bone
Forecannon
Sesamoid
Pedal bone
Long pastern bone
Short pastern bone

Due to its large size and weight, the skeletal system is prone to injury, particularly in the limbs, joints and spine. Injuries such as fractures and joint damage can be devastating to a horse's health and ability to perform and can be challenging to treat and manage. Additionally, certain conformational defects or abnormalities in the skeletal structure can lead to poor performance or chronic health issues.

As discussed in Chapter 1, although horses were not intended to be ridden, they are often expected to perform rigorous athletic activities while carrying a rider, which can lead to injuries. However, horse owners can help reduce the risk of injury and improve performance by implementing proper exercise routines, utilising manual therapy and ensuring optimal management practices. By taking these measures,

owners can effectively prevent or decrease injuries and promote better performance in their horses.

SKELETAL ANATOMY SIMPLIFIED

The horse's skeletal system, comprised of 205 bones, provides essential support and protection for the animal's body, allowing for incredible speed and agility while also supporting its enormous weight. It is divided into the axial skeleton, which supports the head, neck and torso, and the appendicular skeleton, responsible for the horse's limb movement. The skeletal anatomy includes long and flexible neck vertebrae, a relatively rigid back, a short and wide pelvis for powerful muscle attachment and fore and hind limbs with ball and socket joints for a wide range of

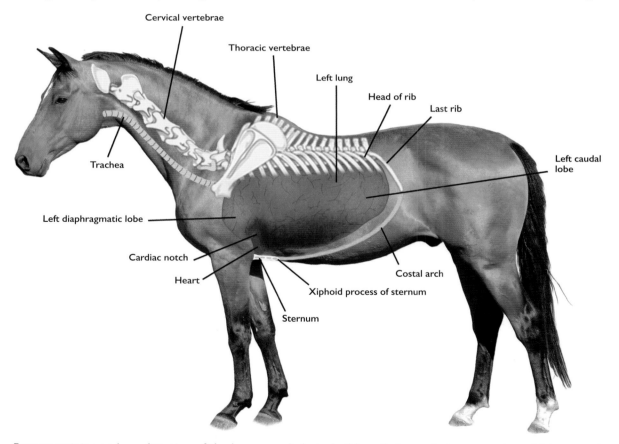

Cervical vertebrae

Thoracic vertebrae

Left lung

Head of rib

Last rib

Left caudal lobe

Trachea

Left diaphragmatic lobe

Cardiac notch

Heart

Xiphoid process of sternum

Costal arch

Sternum

Proper training and conditioning of the horse can help to build up their respiratory muscles, which can make it easier for them to breathe even when carrying a rider. Time spent in flexion should be limited, as this has been shown to restrict the airways and supply of vital oxygen to muscles.

motion. The horse's feet are protected by a keratinous hoof wall, with bones arranged to provide support and stability for weight-bearing and joint movement.

THE HORSE'S SPINE

The horse's spine, also known as the vertebral column, plays several vital roles in its body. The spine supports the weight of the horse's body and helps it maintain balance whilst standing and moving. Although the saddle and rider do not sit directly on the horse's spinal cord, it is a delicate and important structure that runs along the horse's spine and is responsible for transmitting nerve impulses between the brain and the rest of the body. The saddle must be fitted and positioned correctly to avoid pressure or injury to the horse's spine, spinal cord and back muscles. Also, the rider should be symmetrical and not carry any injuries for which the horse's back will make compensation in its movement.

The spine and ribs are also responsible for the movement of the rib cage, which is necessary for breathing. When a rider sits on a horse's back, their weight can compress the horse's lungs and make it more difficult for the horse to breathe. This can be especially problematic with a heavier rider or during intense physical activity, such as galloping, jumping or dressage, when the horse's respiratory system is already working harder to supply oxygen to the muscles. Riders must be aware of this and try to distribute their weight evenly on the horse's back to minimise the amount of compression on the lungs. Any injury or disease that affects the spine can cause serious problems, such as lameness, chronic pain and reduced mobility and performance.

BONE MATURITY

Bone maturity is an essential factor to consider in training horses. A horse's bones reach maturity at around five years of age, and before that, their bones are still growing and developing. During this time, horses are more susceptible to injuries and damage

★ **TOP TIP**

Every horse is different, and some may have pre-existing conditions due to training methods or genetic predispositions that make them more susceptible to bone and joint problems. When acquiring an ex-racehorse, showjumper or any horse that started its career early, make sure you are prepared for the likelihood that it will need careful management in terms of its bone and joint health and extra diligence during exercise, as you may inherit a horse with weakness or injury and even degeneration such as osteoarthritis. This can be seen as early as two years of age in some racehorses. You would need to be prepared for regular veterinary check-ups and preventative measures such as joint supplements, joint injections or other treatments that can be offered by musculoskeletal therapists, such as electrotherapies and kinesiology taping.

from repetitive or excessive stress. This is why we see many injuries in racehorses and other disciplines due to the demands placed on horses at a young age. Over-training, intense exercise, or training too early in a horse's life can result in premature wear and tear on the bones and joints, leading to injuries such as stress fractures, bone chips or degenerative joint disease.

Therefore, it is imperative to gradually introduce exercise and training to horses as their bones develop and mature, avoiding intense and high-impact activities that could cause harm. It is also important to provide a balanced diet with adequate calcium and phosphorus to support proper bone growth. Proper training techniques, including gradual progression, conditioning and rest periods, can help minimise the risk of injury and promote healthy bone development. If any potential issues are suspected, professional help must be sought and addressed promptly.

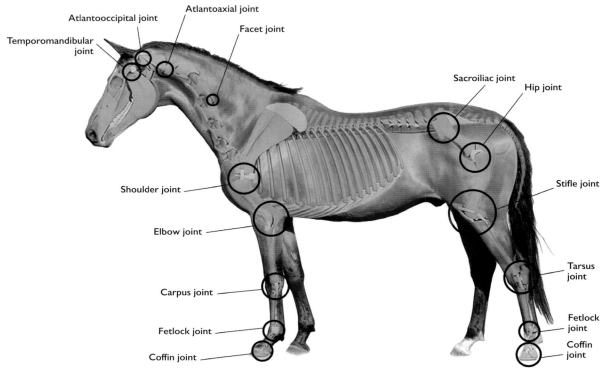

Proper nutrition is important for joint health, as certain vitamins and minerals, such as vitamin C and copper, are necessary for cartilage and joint tissue development and maintenance.

JOINTS

Horses have a variety of joints throughout their body, which allow for movement and flexibility in the limbs, as well as stability and support for the horse's body weight. Proper care of a horse's joints is important for maintaining overall health and performance. This includes correct exercise and conditioning to keep the joints strong and flexible and to avoid excessive strain or stress on the joints. Correct farriery is also essential, including balancing the feet.

The horses' joints are at risk, with horses engaged in high-impact activities such as jumping or racing. It is also important to provide comfortable and supportive schooling and turnout surfaces to reduce the risk of concussion and joint injuries.

The Muscular System

The horse's muscular system comprises a complex network of muscles, tendons and ligaments that allow the horse to move, maintain balance and posture, and perform various physical tasks. It is made up of over 600 muscles that are responsible for movement and body control. The horse's muscles are highly developed, allowing them to move quickly and with great agility. These qualities are largely due to the intricate anatomy and functioning of their muscles; they have a unique combination of slow-twitch and fast-twitch muscle fibres that allow them to perform a wide range of physical activities, from sprinting to endurance.

The complex network of muscles works together for movement and stability. The neck muscles are responsible for the movement and flexion of the neck and play a crucial role in stabilising the head and neck during movement. The back muscles are essential in supporting the rider's weight and evenly distributing it across the horse's back, as well as controlling the movement of the horse's spine. The shoulder muscles assist in the movement of the shoulder joint and stabilise the shoulder blade during movement. The hindquarter muscles are responsible for the propulsion and drive of the horse and help stabilise the hindquarters during movement. The abdominal muscles play a role in stabilising the horse's trunk during movement and support and control the horse's back and hindquarters. Lastly, the limb muscles are responsible for the movement and control of the horse's legs, as well as the coordination and balance required for locomotion.

Supporting their muscular system is a highly developed respiratory system that helps to supply muscles with oxygen. Horses' lungs are large and efficient, allowing them to take in large amounts of air and extract oxygen more effectively. This helps to ensure that their muscles receive the oxygen they need to perform at their best.

Also, they have an excellent cardiovascular system that helps to distribute oxygen and nutrients to their muscles. Their heart is powerful and efficient, and it can pump large amounts of blood to their muscles quickly and efficiently. This helps to ensure that their muscles have the energy they need to perform at their best.

Proper care and exercise are essential for maintaining the health and function of the horse's muscular system.

Proper training and conditioning of both sets of muscles can help prevent pain and injury, promote balance and improve the horse's performance. Targeting superficial and deep muscles achieves a well-rounded, balanced and athletic horse. This is covered in Chapter 8 because a common problem for horses is that superficial muscles are well trained.

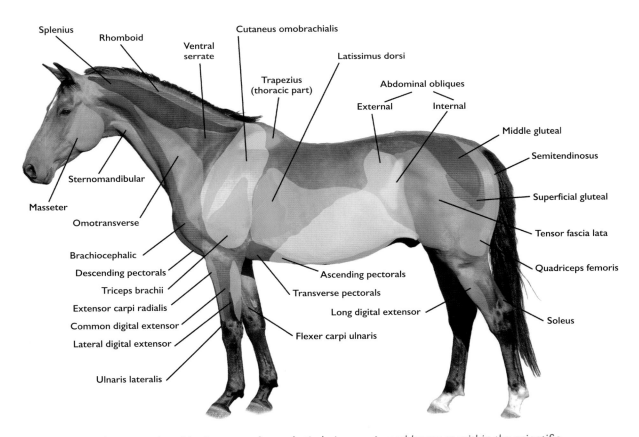

Superficial muscles are assigned Latin names due to Latin being a universal language within the scientific community, enabling therapists, veterinarians, and anatomists to communicate clearly and consistently, regardless of their native language. Slight variations in names may be observed across different reference materials.

In contrast, underlying deep muscles lack strength, so when the horse has an injury or weakness in the superficial muscles, it cannot call on the deep muscles for support because they are also weak; this is when a further injury occurs, and performance fails.

MUSCLE STRUCTURE AND FUNCTION

Muscles are composed of fibres, which are made up of myofibrils, which in turn are composed of myofilaments. Muscle fibres contain both actin and myosin, the proteins that allow muscles to contract and relax. They work in pairs and also in groups of pairs and chains. When one muscle contracts, it becomes shorter, the opposing muscle relaxes and lengthens, which allows for smooth and coordinated movement, also called the agonist-antagonist muscle pair.

MUSCLE INFORMATION PROCESSING

This refers to how the nervous system receives, interprets and responds to information from the muscles, an example of how body systems work together. Sensory receptors in the muscles, called muscle spindles, detect muscle length and tension changes. These receptors send signals to the spinal cord, where interneurons process them. The spinal cord then sends signals, in the form of motor neurons, to the muscles to cause a response. The response can be a reflexive action, such as a stretch reflex, which helps to maintain muscle tone and prevent injury, or a voluntary action, such as the movement of a limb.

The motor neurons also send signals back to the spinal cord and brain to update the sensory information; this process is called proprioception. The brain also receives signals from other senses, such as vision and balance, to coordinate the movements and fine-tune the muscle's response.

Muscle information processing is a complex process involving the coordination of many different parts of the nervous system. As a result, it plays a crucial role in the body's ability to move and function.

SUPERFICIAL AND DEEP MUSCLES

The distinction between superficial and deep muscles in a horse's skeletal system is based on their location in relation to the surface of the horse's body. Superficial muscles are those located closer to the skin and are often large and easily palpated. They are responsible for the horse's visible shape and form, as well as its movement, balance, and posture. These muscles are also called the movement or gymnastic muscles.

In contrast, deep muscles are located further beneath the surface, closer to the bone, and play a more supportive role in maintaining the horse's overall muscular structure and function; these cannot be palpated. Understanding the difference between superficial and deep muscles is important for proper training, conditioning and care of the horse's muscular system.

DORSAL CHAIN (EXTENSOR CHAIN)

These refer to the superficial and deep muscles along the body's top line (dorsal). These are mainly responsible for the extension of the spine, which enables the horse to stretch and reach further with its legs, resulting in longer and more powerful strides. This chain also provides stability for the forelimbs, helping maintain balance and coordination while moving.

VENTRAL CHAIN (FLEXOR CHAIN)

These refer to the superficial and deep muscles on the horse's hip flexor and the abdominal and thoracic regions (ventral). These are mainly responsible for the muscles that flex the elbow and shoulder, which allows the horse to bring its forelimbs closer to its body and perform movements such as collecting and shortening the stride as well as providing support for the forelimbs, propulsion and power, especially when elevating its forelimbs.

Both chains need to be equally as strong so that the horse can support itself in self-carriage, making it stronger and more athletic, which is essential

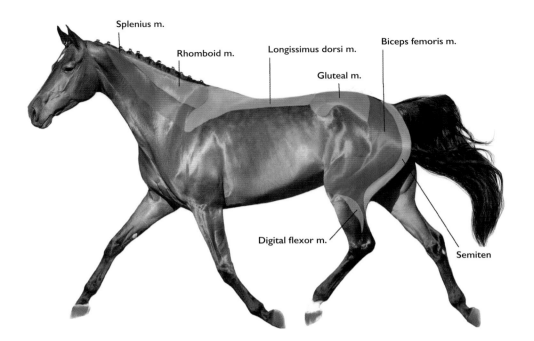

Splenius m.

Rhomboid m.

Longissimus dorsi m.

Gluteal m.

Biceps femoris m.

Digital flexor m.

Semiten

Propulsion and power are key features of this chain to propel the horse forward, especially in faster gaits and jumping.

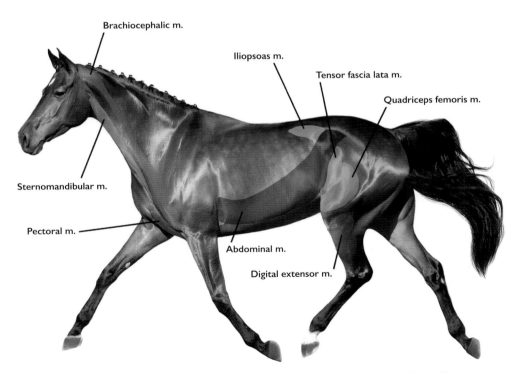

Brachiocephalic m.

Iliopsoas m.

Tensor fascia lata m.

Quadriceps femoris m.

Sternomandibular m.

Pectoral m.

Abdominal m.

Digital extensor m.

When the horse moves, the dorsal chain extends, whereas the ventral chain flexes. This allows you to see how important it is for the horse to engage its core, which helps lift and lengthen the back.

for any equestrian discipline from dressage to horseracing. A disruption in the chains is often seen when the abdominals drop and pull the back into a hollow position; this is a weakness.

MUSCLE BALANCE

Achieving correct muscle balance in a horse can be challenging due to several reasons. Horses carry most of their weight naturally on the forehand because their head and neck are relatively heavy compared to the rest of their body. Additionally, when a horse moves, its front legs reach out farther and strike the ground with more force than its hind legs, contributing to the weight being shifted to the forehand. The shape and angle of the horse's spine and pelvis are

★ **TOP TIP**

Equestrians often assume that their horse is well balanced at first glance, but a more critical assessment or a professional therapist's opinion may reveal areas of tension or weakness in the horse's body. It is important to evaluate your horse while standing without any tack and while moving without a rider. By closely observing the horse's muscles, one can gain valuable insight into their physical condition. Conducting a comprehensive examination of your horse can unveil crucial information that might otherwise be missed but is essential for their overall health and progress.

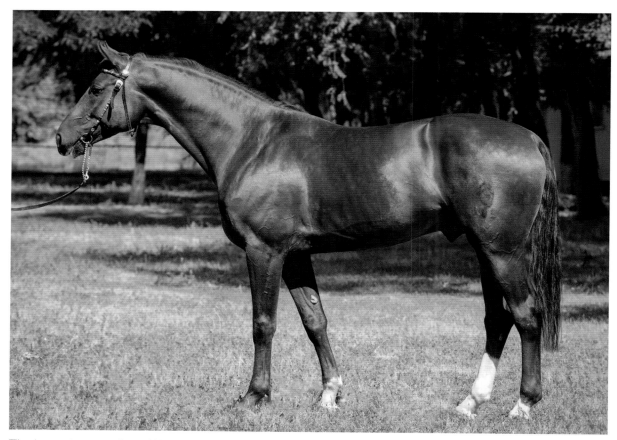

The horse is generally well balanced and has well-developed muscles, although tension in the upper middle section of the neck is noticeable. Likely caused by incorrect bit or bridle, rigid rider hands or training aids. Tension will affect the horse's balance and motion; manual therapy can alleviate it.

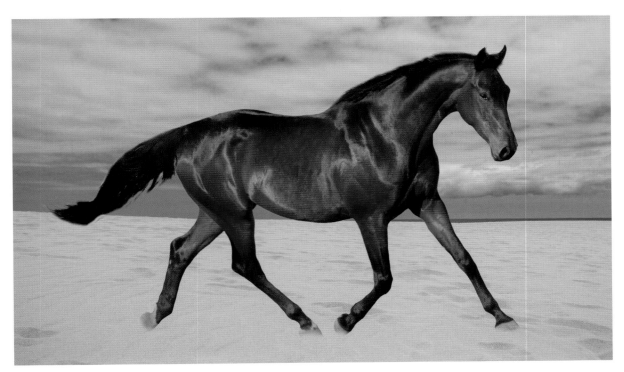

The horse displays balanced movement and freedom of motion without a rider. Its hindquarters are engaged, allowing the hind hoof to step into the forehoof print, while its core is activated, back lifted and front end lifted upward and forward, creating a good position for the head and neck without any tension. This correct use of the body is highly advantageous.

also factors that contribute to weight distribution, as the horse's centre of gravity is located closer to the front of its body. This natural weight distribution can be problematic for the horse, which is why proper training and conditioning are important to develop a more balanced weight distribution, especially crucial when carrying a rider. If the rider is unbalanced, tense or heavy-handed, this can interfere with the horse's ability to move in balance, which results in imbalanced muscle development.

Achieving correct muscle balance in a horse requires a combination of factors, including the horse's natural tendencies, conformation, rider position and fitness. It can take time, patience and expertise to develop a horse's balance and maintain it throughout its training and development. It is very challenging to find a horse that exhibits complete muscle balance without any signs of tension or weakness. I come across very few in the many horses I treat, and this in-

cludes Group One racehorses, Olympians and Grand Prix horses.

Although a well-muscled and balanced horse is preferred and beneficial in every way, it is unfortunately not a common sight in the equine industry at all levels.

A weak and unbalanced horse can be a challenge to ride and train. It may lack muscle tone and strength in key areas, such as the hindquarters, back and core, leading to difficulty maintaining balance and proper posture. This can result in a choppy or uncoordinated gait, with the horse struggling to move fluidly and efficiently. In addition, an unbalanced horse may have difficulty responding to cues and may be prone to stumbling or tripping, which can be dangerous for both the rider and the horse. Proper training and conditioning can help improve the horse's muscle tone and balance, but it requires patience, consistency, and a skilled rider to bring the horse to a level of fitness

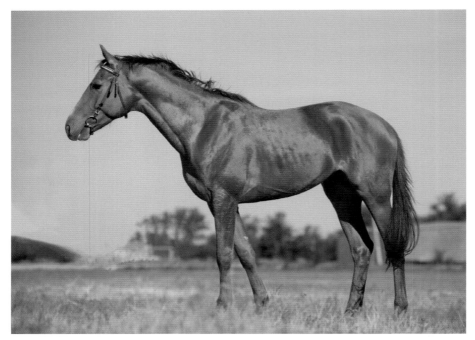

The horse is weak and unbalanced, showing tension in the upper neck, likely due to incorrect equipment, rider's hands or training aids. It has some shoulder muscling but still exhibits tension. The back, core and hindquarters are weak with atrophy, with evidence of tension. This horse tends to lean on the forehand and lacks engagement of the hindquarters. It is a common yet undesirable sight in horses.

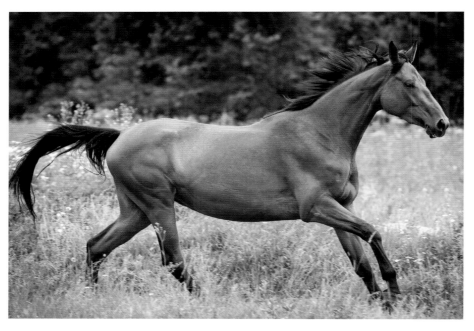

This horse is unbalanced and weak in motion, relying on its neck to compensate for its lack of strength and balance. Its back shows signs of atrophy and is hollow, indicating weakness and its core and hindquarters also appear weak. It uses its tail to assist with balance. As a result, the horse is moving on the forehand without proper engagement from the hindquarters.

where it can move with ease and grace.

A horse with a downwardly extended topline and a hollow back is not moving in a balanced and efficient manner. The horse may carry its head and neck high while lacking engagement of the core and hindquarters, resulting in a heavy forehand. As a result, the horse's legs may not track up correctly. This type of movement can strain the ligaments of the hind legs, which may become over-stretched due to the tilting forward of the pelvis and also can cause the vertebrae in the back to become closer together, leading to potential pain and issues with spinal health.

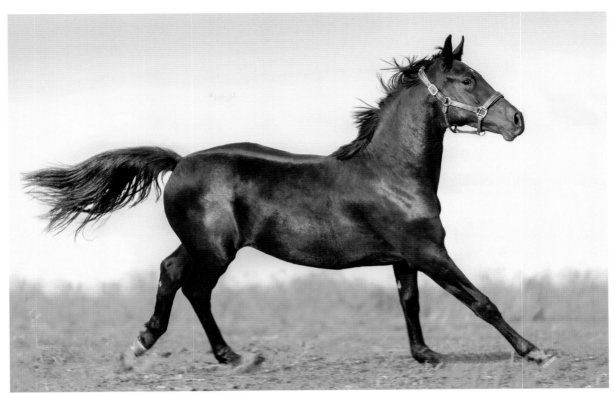

This horse's downwardly extended topline creates an imbalance; there is no hindquarter engagement or tracking up. It is leaning on the inside forelimb and hindlimb, increasing the risk of injury. A high head and hollow back show clear tension lines with shoulder and forelimb reduced range of motion. A horse moving in this way freely is unlikely to move in engagement with a rider unless it is forced, which is an unwelcome sight and very damaging.

MUSCLE CONDITIONS AND INJURIES

Muscle conditions and injuries can be any damage or harm that affects the horse's muscles and their ability to function normally. These occur mainly due to incorrect exercise, riding styles, repetitive strain and accidents. Common muscle injuries include:

Strains – these occur when muscle fibres are stretched or torn due to overstretching, overuse or overloading the muscle. They are common in the back, hamstring and neck muscles.

Contusions – also known as bruises. A contusion occurs when a muscle is hit hard enough to cause blood vessels to rupture, leading to bleeding, localised pain and sometimes swelling. Examples include that caused by an incorrect fitting saddle bruising the spine, especially if the saddle moves because it is unstable, the rider mounts from the ground, or the channel is too narrow. A contusion can also occur when the horse rolls on a stone in the paddock or knocks itself when entering or exiting the stable, field, etc. These can take up to several weeks to repair.

Tears – are when muscle fibres are completely ruptured, usually associated with severe pain and weakness.

Sprains – this happens when the muscle is stretched or torn from the attachment site on the bone, which is the ligament. Sprains most commonly occur in the horse's knee (carpus), fetlock and hock (tarsus).

Tendinitis – this is inflammation of the tendons that attach muscle to bone, caused by overuse and repetitive motions.

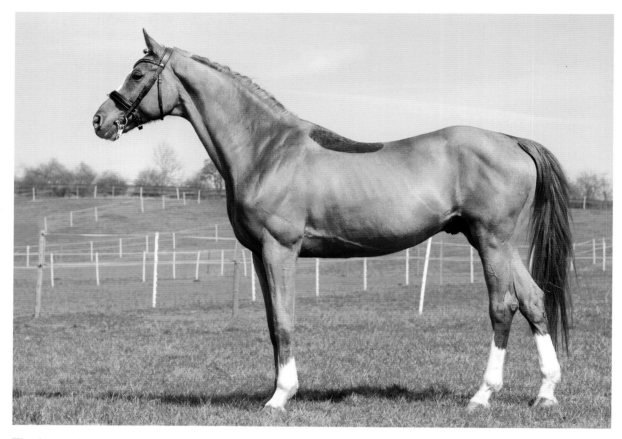

This horse shows signs of atrophy in several muscle groups, including the neck, back, hip flexors and gluteal muscles, as well as muscle tension that may result from improper training aids. The horse may be working in an overbent manner, likely with side reins, which is not promoting healthy muscle development or movement.

The symptoms of muscle injuries may include pain, weakness, muscle spasms, adhesions, swelling and tenderness. Depending on the severity of the injury, it might require rest and cryotherapy (such as cold compressing or hosing) and gentle manual therapy, as it heals with a gradual return to work.

When the horse is continually being exercised incorrectly, it can lead to unfavourable muscle conditions such as muscle atrophy, hypertonicity and asymmetry, all commonly seen by musculo-skeletal therapists when attending to horses in our clinical work.

Muscle Atrophy

This is a condition which is the wasting or loss of muscle mass and strength. A variety of factors – such as disuse, misuse, ageing, poor nutrition, hormonal imbalances, neurological conditions and certain medical conditions – can cause it. Symptoms of muscle atrophy include a decrease in muscle mass, weakness and difficulty performing tasks. Manual therapy is a positive way to increase blood flow to the atrophied muscles and start the regeneration process with correct supportive exercise.

When horses are seen with a disruption to their dorsal and ventral chain, they are unbalanced, and there is a weakness in the muscles that connect the front and back of the horse's body. As well as a lack of coordination in movement, this weakness can lead to compensatory movement patterns that can result in muscle tension and atrophy, as well as other issues

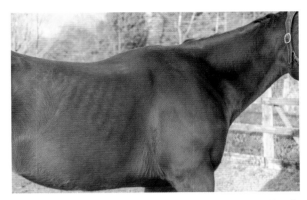

This horse has atrophy to its neck, withers and back. The dorsal and ventral chains are disrupted and, therefore, weak. The horse is a thoroughbred with a large frame, but its muscles are atrophied to the extent that there is little support for its skeleton. It would require correct supportive exercise comprising in-hand work only until he became stronger to support himself, before carrying a rider.

such as joint pain or stiffness.

Muscle Hypertrophy

Muscle hypertrophy is a condition that refers to an increase in the size and mass of the horse's muscles due to the growth and multiplication of muscle fibres. This process occurs in response to physical activity or exercises that stress the muscles beyond their normal capacity, such as consistent training or work, as with racehorses and other competing equine athletes. Hypertrophy results in the muscles being stronger and more resilient.

In horses, muscle hypertrophy can be beneficial, as it allows the horse to perform better, become more athletic and handle greater physical demands without experiencing fatigue. It can also improve the horse's overall health and wellbeing by increasing its metabolism and reducing the risk of obesity and other health issues.

It is important to note that muscle hypertrophy is achieved through a well-planned and gradual training programme to prevent overloading the horse's muscles, which it would then be deemed as a negative whilst causing hypertonicity, injury or strain. Proper nutrition, rest and recovery are also important.

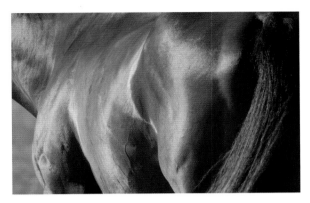

An increase in muscle definition gives the appearance of looking more toned and athletic, but without tension lines or surrounding atrophy.

Muscle Hypertonicity

Hypertonicity is a condition in which muscles have excessive tone and remain contracted, even when they are at rest. This condition can arise due to various factors such as overtraining, incorrect training, use of training aids, muscle strain or injury. Hypertonicity can cause stiffness, pain and reduced range of motion, and often requires manual therapy to gently stretch and loosen the affected muscle, and increase circulation. It is essential to modify the horse's exercise routine to prevent the recurrence of this condition.

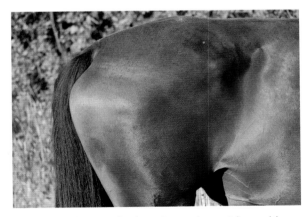

This horse has weak gluteal muscles, evidenced by the lack of round shaping from the croup to the tail; there is too much slope and insufficient muscle and also underdeveloped hip flexors. A slight dip in front of the croup indicates incorrect pelvic movement, as do the hamstrings, which are overdeveloped with hypertonicity.

Hypertonicity may not be easily identifiable by an untrained therapist and can lead to numerous issues if left untreated, such as chronic pain, muscle imbalances, limited mobility and even the risk of tearing. It is crucial to address this issue as soon as possible to avoid further complications.

Muscle Asymmetry

This is a situation where the muscles on one side of the body are not the same size or strength as those on the other. This can occur due to various factors, including injury, disease, overuse, misuse, unlevel rider or saddle or simply the horse favouring one side over the other. Improper training, saddle damage, unlevel riders and lack of turnout are the common causes. Asymmetry affects balance and movement as well as pain and discomfort for the horse.

Assessing a horse's muscles from the rear is advantageous, as it offers a clear perspective on muscle symmetry and balance. The hindquarters of a horse house some of the largest and most powerful muscles, which play a vital role in movement and overall performance.

When observed from behind, a horse's muscles should exhibit symmetry on both sides of the body. Any signs of asymmetry or unevenness in the muscles may indicate an underlying issue, such as muscle at-

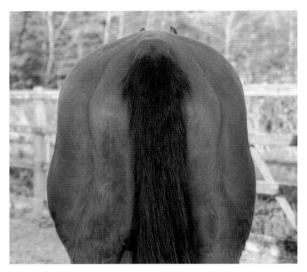

This horse's hamstring muscle group exhibits asymmetry, potentially resulting from various factors, including incorrect exercise techniques that fail to engage the hindquarters evenly, injury or overuse of one side leading to uneven muscle development, favouring one leg and working predominantly on one side, and certain conditions like lameness and osteoarthritis, contributing to muscle imbalances.

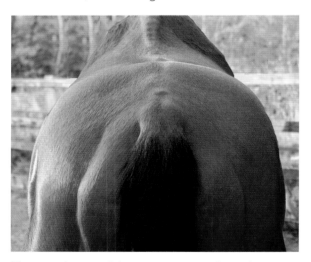

The same horse exhibits asymmetry in the withers, with significant differences, along with a rightward curve in the thoracic spine. The left hind is more developed than the right, suggesting an imbalance. These findings indicate a potential issue with the saddle fit, hindering shoulder movement and possibly causing spinal damage from injury or improper fit. The asymmetry between the front and hind suggests overall crookedness in the horse, likely from an injury that was not rehabilitated.

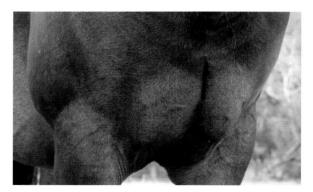

This horse has asymmetry in its pectoral muscles in the chest. Primarily responsible for flexing and extending the shoulder and assisting in lateral movements such as turning and bending and also front limb movement. The horse's skin looks very dry, which could indicate dehydration or poor circulation.

rophy, hypertonicity or injury. Once such asymmetry is identified, a targeted treatment plan becomes necessary to address the problem effectively. This can involve various approaches, including manual therapy and correct supportive exercises to target specific areas of weakness and promote balanced muscle development. Additionally, the application of kinesiology taping techniques can prove beneficial in addressing asymmetry.

Assessing the asymmetry of muscles alongside a horse's spine can help to identify potential issues, such as incorrect saddle fit, vertebral misalignments or muscle strains. For example, if one side of the muscling alongside the spine is more developed, it could be a sign of uneven pressure distribution or compensation from an injury. The development of these muscles also depends on the horse's exercise regime, so a lack of development on one side could indicate poor training techniques or uneven use of the horse's body during exercise or if compensating for an unlevel rider.

It is worth noting that some degree of asymmetry is normal in horses, as they tend to have a dominant side. However, significant or progressive asymmetry should be monitored and addressed to prevent potential complications.

An excellent way to check asymmetry is to use a flexi curve, which you can bend over the horse's

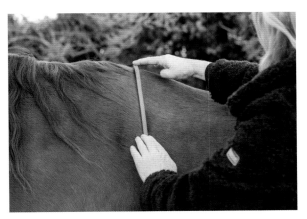

A flexi curve is placed over the horse's withers and moulded to the shape to create a template.

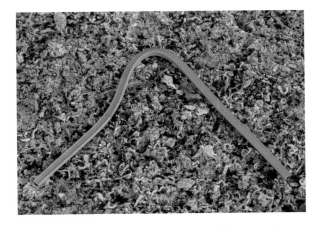

The template of the flexi curve identifies atrophy to the left side of the horse's withers, which indicates that the saddle has been pinching the horse here.

withers or other areas of the spine and hindquarters to give you an impression, take a photograph of that and date it, which will be the benchmark before you start your treatment plan. Periodically you can repeat this and monitor the change in the horse's shape.

Connective Tissue

Connective tissue is a diverse group of tissues in the body that provides support and protection to the body and is involved in many functions, such as repair and regeneration, immune response and homeostasis. There are several types including:

Loose connective tissue – this includes areolar and adipose tissue. Areolar tissue is found in various parts of the body, such as around blood vessels and nerves, and is composed of fibres and ground substance, a gelatinous material. It is transparent and fills the spaces between fibres and cells. Adipose tissue is made up of fat cells and is found under the skin and around organs.

Dense connective tissue – this includes tendons, ligaments and fascia. Tendons are composed of dense regular connective tissue and attach muscle to bone. Ligaments are composed of dense regular connective tissue and connect bone to bone.

Specialised connective tissue – this includes cartilage, bone, and blood. Cartilage is a type of connective tissue that provides support and cushioning in joints; bone provides support and protection for the body; and blood carries oxygen and nutrients to the body's cells.

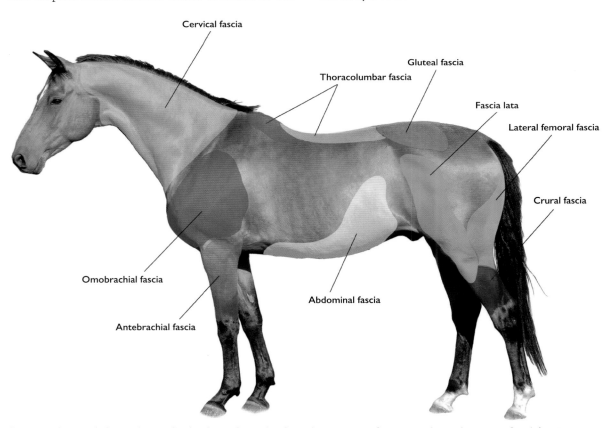

Fascia is located throughout the body and can be found in various forms, such as the superficial fascia shown in the image (just under the skin), deep fascia (around muscles and organs), and visceral fascia (around internal organs).

All forms of connective tissue play a vital role in preserving the horse's body, ensuring its structural integrity, and maintaining optimal functional capacity. When it comes to tendon or ligament injuries, expert care is essential to facilitate the best possible healing process.

FASCIA

Fascia, consisting of fibrous tissue comprising collagen, elastin and other fibres, serves several crucial functions in the horse's body. It provides structural support, facilitates movement and flexibility, enables effective force transmission among muscles, and protects the body's organs and nerves from potential injuries.

Myofascial release is a manual therapy technique designed to target and address the fascia throughout the horse's body. By focusing on the fascia, myofascial release helps promote optimal function and wellbeing.

It is worth noting that scientific research has emphasised the significance of fascia in healing injuries and addressing chronic pain. Various therapies, including myofascial release, are being used to target fascial restrictions in the body to help alleviate pain and improve function.

As an expert in musculoskeletal therapy, I incorporate myofascial release in my practice, and this book also covers this powerful modality. It is worth mentioning that I was one of the first to perform equine myofascial release several years ago when it was still in the early stages of human research. Today, it has become widely accepted as an effective approach in equine musculoskeletal therapy.

THE EQUINE FOOT

The equine foot – also known as the horse's hoof – is a crucial anatomical part; it is a complex structure that plays a critical role in the horse's ability to move and support its weight. Proper hoof care is essential for the horse's overall health and well-being, as well-maintained hooves can also help prevent lameness in the feet, limbs and the upper body.

★ **TOP TIP**

I always conduct a thorough inspection of the horse's feet, as it provides valuable information about how the horse will support its body and move. One common problem I have encountered is when a horse has one foot with a high heel and the other with a low heel, as I referred to in Chapter 1. The front foot with the high heel can create tension in the limb and shoulder, while the low heel can cause weakness in the tendons and ligaments of the limb. When this imbalance occurs in the hind feet pair, it can lead to hock and pelvic problems, affecting the horse's strength and balance.

Over the years, I have witnessed numerous tendon and ligament injuries in horses, particularly in the limb with the low heel. In fact, based on my observations, I am confident in saying that high heel and low heel imbalances can cause horses to break down entirely, often causing severe ligament injuries in the limb with the low heel. Therefore, it is crucial to address any such issues early on to prevent potential injuries and ensure the horse's optimal health and performance. If your farrier is unable to assist, then find one who can.

Of extreme importance is hoof balance, which is the alignment and proportion of various parts of the hoof, including the hoof wall, sole, frog, heel and digital cushion, in relation to the horse's limb and body.

Proper hoof balance is essential for the following reasons:

Weight-bearing and support – this allows the horse to distribute its weight evenly across the entire hoof, which helps to prevent overloading and damage to any one part of the hoof. This is especially important for horses used for heavy work or performance activities.

Movement and gait – a balanced hoof allows the

horse to move and walk with a natural gait, which helps to prevent injuries and lameness. An unbalanced hoof can cause the horse to move unevenly, leading to strain on the joints, tendons and ligaments and problems such as navicular disease. Many horses present with navicular disease but have never received a diagnosis.

Traction and stability – a balanced hoof provides the horse with better traction and stability, which is especially important for horses ridden or used for activities on uneven terrain such as eventing or hunting, helping to prevent slips and falls, which can be dangerous for the horse and rider.

Pain and discomfort – an unbalanced hoof can cause pain and discomfort for the horse, which can affect its overall wellbeing and behaviour, which can lead to a decrease in performance and an increase in stress-related behaviours such as crib-biting and other stereotypies.

Longevity – a balanced hoof can help to prolong the life of the horse's hoof by preventing overuse, trauma and chronic conditions from occurring.

Equine Dentition

Correct equine dentition is critical in the horse's ability to chew and digest food. Therefore, proper dental care is essential for the horse's overall health and wellbeing, as poor dental health can lead to difficulty eating, weight loss and other health problems.

Sharp edges on teeth reduce chewing efficiency and interfere with jaw motion and, in extreme cases, can cut the tongue or cheek, making eating and riding painful for the horse. This is why it is important for regular dental examinations by a well-qualified equine dentist or equine veterinarian trained in dentistry. A horse's teeth should be checked at least annually. However, best practice would be every six months, to keep teeth and the chewing action in optimum condition.

In the wild, a horse's teeth wear differently than in domestication because natural foodstuffs would allow teeth to wear more evenly. Because many modern horses often graze on lusher, softer forage than their wild ancestors, and are also frequently fed grain or other concentrated feed, natural wear may be reduced in the domestic horse.

Evidence is now suggesting that concentrated feed is bad for the horse's teeth due to the high content of sugar and the shaping of the feed that can get impacted between the horse's teeth, causing problems such as tooth decay and gum disease.

THE BIT

When fitting a bit to a horse, the metal bar of the bit should be positioned correctly in the interdental space between the incisors and premolars. Poorly adjusted bridles can cause the bit to rest too low or high, resulting in discomfort and exacerbating any pre-existing dental or oral cavity conformation issues the horse may have.

A well-fitted bit enables the rider to communicate clearly and consistently with the horse, improving responsiveness and performance while also preventing resistance and promoting balance. However, proper

> ### ★ TOP TIP
> I have encountered cases where horses display unresponsiveness to the bit, difficulty with steering, leaning to one side and also exhibiting symptoms such as nasal discharge, facial swelling and foul breath, which often indicate dental problems. Unfortunately, some owners fail to notice these. Dental problems such as impactions and fractures can cause significant pain to the horse, and in one instance, I encountered a horse whose tooth was so sharp that it was digging into its cheek. The use of a flash noseband by the rider only added to the horse's pain, resulting in it rearing up. In that instance, I was contacted to check the horse's back. Inadequate basic management is often the cause of such problems.

bit fitting is a complex process that takes into account various factors, such as mouth conformation, tongue size and the horse's preferences regarding tongue pressure or bar pressure. Seeking the advice of a bit-fitting expert or completing my online course can help ensure proper bit selection and fitting.

Inadequate bit and bridle fitting, dental problems and rough rider hands can cause pain in the horse's muscular system around its skull, leading to severe musculoskeletal issues, behavioural problems and loss of performance if not addressed. Therefore, it is essential to examine the horse's teeth, bit and headgear when it is exhibiting any behavioural or performance-related problems.

TMJ (TEMPOROMANDIBULAR JOINT)

In anatomy, this joint connects the horse's skull to the lower jaw. Its primary function is to allow the horse to move its jaw up and down and side to side for chewing and grinding food. The TMJ is a complex joint that is made up of several different parts, including the temporal bone, the mandible and the articular disc.

Problems with the horse's TMJ can lead to pain and difficulty eating, as well as other issues such as difficulty opening the jaw, difficulty closing the jaw, or even difficulty with facial expressions, sensitivity around the area, the ears and head shyness. Often the problems are due to the horse tugging on hay nets, being ridden in too much flexion, incorrect bit, heavy rider hands, locking the head into position with training aids and poor dental care. Many horses are

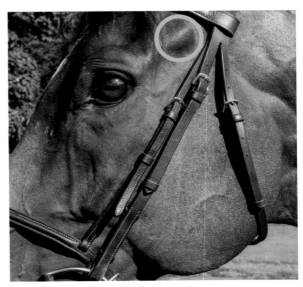

The TMJ is indicated by the yellow circle.

diagnosed with disease or osteoarthritis of the TMJ, and I suspect many have it but go undiagnosed. Researchers in Canada found that TMJ inflammation causes rein lameness in horses.

Ensure the bridle is clear of the TMJ; I have seen many buckle fastenings situated too close to the TMJ, causing abrasion and inflammation. Ergonomic or anatomical bridles are, in my opinion, the best: they are designed to be comfortable for the horse and to relieve pressure on the skull. Every piece is shaped and positioned, considering the bones, nerves, tendons, ligaments and contours of the horse's head. When the horse is more comfortable, it can focus on its schooling instead of the pressure and pain from a bridle or bit.

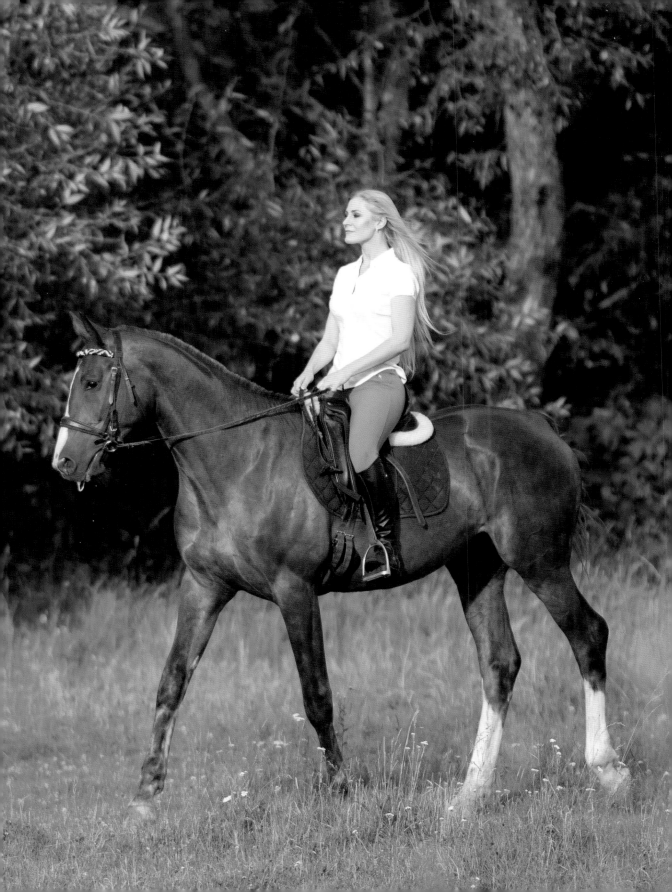

CHAPTER 4

Training, Performance and Musculoskeletal Health

To avoid pain and injury, the training of horses must be tailored to their individual needs, as each horse possesses distinctive physical traits, abilities and limitations. Thus, a standardised approach to exercise and training is not feasible or effective for all horses. A customised programme can cater to the horse's particular requirements, consider its distinctive traits, and help rectify any issues or imbalances. Consequently, this can enhance performance and minimise the risk of musculoskeletal pain and injury to enhance the overall welfare of the horse.

Horses have unique physical adaptations that make them great athletes, but also more prone to injury. To ensure the best outcomes for horses, a team approach with a willingness to learn and try new methods is essential. Unfortunately, many horses do not reach their full potential because their training is not tailored to their individual needs or is unrealistic, resulting in rushed progress and injuries.

Training and Performance

It is important to understand the different categories of training and where the horse should be at all times, taking into account factors such as the horse's age, current fitness, health, conformation and any previous injuries. Competition goals should not dictate the horse's training; instead, the horse's preparation and readiness must come first before any competition is considered. Unfortunately, some people prioritise their own desire to compete over the horse's wellbeing.

During the training process, setbacks, progress and modifications to training are expected, as horses are living mammals and athletes. We will cover in this chapter specific riding styles that can influence muscle health, pain and injury, as well as the various training categories, including pre-training, strength and conditioning training, continuation training, rehabilitation and warm-up and cool-down protocols.

During all stages of training, it is important to allow the horse specific periods of rest, since training can be physically and mentally demanding for them. This is where manual therapy can help, as it provides an excellent opportunity for the horse to relax and shift into parasympathetic mode, away from the pressure of learning. Additionally, this allows you to evaluate the horse's muscles and see how they respond to the training. Ensure you include your manual therapy sessions in the horse's training schedule.

PAIN AND INJURY, CAUSE AND EFFECT

I have already discussed the benefits of manual therapy in Chapter 2 without directly referencing injury cause and effect.

When a horse owner contacts a professional to assist their horse, it is usually because the horse displays symptoms such as reduced performance, a behaviour change, reacting to tack, rearing, bolting and inability to use certain parts of its body as it once did, and so on. These are examples of the effects of an injury that might be new or has been developing over a long period.

It is not the fault of horse owners if they do not always recognise when a problem is manifesting; it is because they are not looking for one. A well-trained musculoskeletal therapist will know the signs to look for and should make it their prime focus to help find the root cause and provide therapy accordingly. The pain and injury's cause and effect will continue if this does not happen, and the longer this continues, the more challenging it is to help the horse. An example of this is a high-level competition horse that appears to be doing well and, from nowhere, it breaks down because something has been building up and going unnoticed. In other cases, horse owners see niggles such as intermittent lameness, and there is always a reason behind it that needs finding. Some causes are easier than others to discover, and in some cases, veterinary diagnostics are required.

Common Causes of Pain and Injury

Other than direct musculoskeletal injuries from accidents, falls, competitive strain and so on, common causes of pain that are often overlooked are:

- The tack is incorrect for the horse.
- Equipment such as training aids are unsuitable and unnecessary for the horse.
- Inadequate farrier, dental and saddle check regimens. These are management basics.
- Unbalanced riders, either due to inexperience or injury; horses frequently compensate in their bodies for rider faults.
- Unsuitable conformation for the equine discipline.
- Previous injuries that have not healed correctly and recur.
- Degeneration in bones and joints.

- Training surfaces that are unsuitable for the horse.
- Inadequate warm-up and cool-down and ridden for too long in flexion or a 'competition frame'.
- Lack of preparation when a horse increases its training and technical skills before its ability and fitness are ready.
- Pushing horses beyond their level.
- Insufficient rest and recovery built into training and competition schedules.
- Not enough time being a horse, grazing with other horses and doing what horses enjoy doing together in a herd.
- Overfeeding and a lack of natural diet that horses' digestive systems crave. Nutrition and feeding are complex, but they do not need to be because the horse's digestive system is basic, and so are its needs.
- Musculoskeletal problems that go unchecked, for which the horse develops compensation patterns causing further injury.
- Stress and anxiety cause immense emotional and physical health issues for horses and can weaken their resilience.

Training for Body Type

It is important to exercise and train a horse in a manner – and ultimately a discipline – that suits its body type, because certain physical characteristics and abilities of the horse are more suited to specific activities.

Horses use their bodies differently based on their breed, conformation and the discipline they are being trained for. Different breeds have been selectively bred for different characteristics and abilities, such as speed, strength, endurance, agility and jumping ability. This leads to variations in their physical conformation, such as the length and angle of their legs, the shape of their hooves and chest and the muscling of their bodies.

Some horses may have physical limitations or injuries that affect how they use their bodies and must be trained and handled accordingly. Training for its body type is essential for optimal performance, preventing injuries and maintaining the horse's health and comfort.

A study on the effects of the EquiAmi™ training aid discovered that it does not have the same effect on every horse, and its effect can vary within the same horse between gaits. Therefore, the individual characteristics and needs of the horse must be considered when applying training aids.

THE THREE MAIN CATEGORIES OF TRAINING

These categories can vary based on the horse's health, fitness, age and the need to prevent recurring injuries. It is important to prioritise the horse's readiness and preparation before focusing on progression through the training categories or specific goals, such as competitions. Rest periods are essential in all training categories to allow the horse's body and mind to recover from training demands. During manual therapy sessions, you can assess how the horse's muscles respond to the training and specific exercises in the programme. In Chapter 8, you will find detailed information on the training categories and exercises to consider for each category.

A correct working frame is a foundation for optimal performance, whether in flatwork or jumping. It enables the horse to maximise its athletic potential, promoting relaxation, suppleness and uphill movement by transferring weight onto the hindquarters.

The First Category is Pre-Training

This initial training phase is advantageous for young horses with developing musculoskeletal systems, preparing them for subsequent strength and conditioning programmes. Rushing or skipping this category will have consequences later in the horse's career, often requiring a return to pre-training as incorrect and premature training can lead to osteoarthritis and other degenerative conditions, commonly observed in racehorses, show jumpers and dressage horses as well as recreational horses.

Pre-training focuses on in-hand exercises such as manoeuvring around cones and obstacles, lunging

without aids to promote the horse's body support, and walking over low poles to enhance proprioception (limb awareness). These exercises help lay a solid foundation for the horse's overall development.

The Second Category is Strength and Conditioning Training

Horses benefit from quality movement achieved through strength and conditioning training, which targets both the deep and superficial muscles. The training in this category aims to improve flexibility, joint range of motion, core engagement, top-line lengthening, stride length and hind limb engagement.

Conditioning training develops the musculoskeletal, neurological and cardiovascular systems, enabling horses to perform athletic activities efficiently and with minimal stress on the body. Pole work, gymnastic jumping exercises, transitions and speed work are some conditioning training examples. Monitoring for signs of body stress, such as muscle soreness, limb swelling, behavioural changes or attitude shifts, is crucial. Palpation, as discussed in Chapter 6, can be a helpful technique.

Strength and conditioning training should be conducted two to three times a week, gradually increasing in intensity every five days. This allows the horse's body to adapt before progressing further while incorporating adequate rest periods into the programmes.

The Third Category is Continuation Training

Once the horse has undergone its pre-training if required – and its strength and conditioning, which is essential for all horses – it should enter the continuation training category. This is an ongoing fitness programme including technical skills, just like any human athlete. This will include a maintenance level of strength and conditioning because the muscles should be maintained to the standard already achieved, and also the learning of more technical skills at given points as it progresses through its dressage or show jumping. It is important not to rush the continuation training; if a horse can easily jump one metre, for example, it does not mean that it should be consistently jumping at this height or moving up to the next height.

OTHER CATEGORIES OF TRAINING

Rehabilitation Training

Rehabilitation training for horses is a different type of training that involves a structured programme of exercise and activities designed to aid in the recovery from injuries or surgeries by rebuilding the horse's strength, flexibility and range of motion, as well as improving their overall fitness level. The training regimen may include a variety of activities, such as walking and trotting on a lunge line, other groundwork exercises tailored to the specific needs and condition of the horse, as well as hydrotherapy under the care of an equine hydrotherapist. Ensure they are trained such as in the online course I offer as, unfortunately, many facilities offer this service, but are not adequately trained in hydrotherapy exercise protocols; as such, this is not a bespoke programme for the horse. The same water height, duration and so on for every horse, can be very damaging, especially if they have injuries that are unknown.

The rehabilitation training plan must be customised to meet the unique needs and conditions of each horse, considering any injury or surgical constraints. This requires the guidance of an experienced mus-

★ TOP TIP

Advice regarding back rehabilitation can vary significantly. Some suggest using training aids to encourage a specific shape, but misuse of such aids can lead to the horse relying on them and working on the forehand instead of achieving self-carriage. This approach does not promote successful back rehabilitation. I recall an incident in which a professional advised strapping a horse's head in with side reins and placing it on a horse walker following surgery, which caused the horse extensive pain and re-injury.

On the other hand, others recommend allowing the horse to naturally learn to engage its back and find balance through exercises such as in-hand work around obstacles and cavaletti. Based on my extensive rehabilitation experience, I have found this approach to be more beneficial. Additionally, allowing the horse regular paddock turnout, in which it can lower its head to graze, promotes natural stretching of the back, which can aid in the rehabilitation process.

Unfortunately, horses cannot verbally express their pain, making it common for people to overlook signs of discomfort during a rehabilitation programme. This oversight can lead to horses struggling to cope, potentially resulting in further injury or a delay in their recovery. Observe your horse's facial expressions and provide regular manual therapy to ensure the best chance of success in the rehabilitation programme.

culoskeletal therapist or veterinarian, depending on the nature of the rehabilitation and the requirements of any insurance company involved. If you are given a rehabilitation activity that seems unclear or concerning to you, it is crucial to ask questions and request an explanation for its rationale.

Recurring Injury Prevention

There are two classes of injuries, traumatic and cumulative. Traumatic injuries are accidents to horses that result in injury or some form of surgery or medical intervention. Cumulative injuries relate to tissue damage over time due to repetitive strain or weakened tissues, such as from wearing an incorrectly fitting saddle, which means the back cannot fully heal, tendon injuries and so on.

If the horse has completed its rehabilitation programme and is now undertaking 'continuation training', it must continually be monitored to prevent a 'recurring injury' – by adjusting the training accordingly and providing manual therapy to support the horse.

Monitoring and Evaluating

Through correct training, balance is achieved, and the horse can move more efficiently and with less strain on its muscles and joints. This can help prevent injuries and prolong the horse's career. A balanced horse can also perform at a higher level in activities such as eventing, jumping and dressage. Additionally, a horse that moves in balance is generally considered more aesthetically pleasing to watch.

The following general guidelines will help you to correctly train your horse:

- Always start with a proper warm-up before any training session; it is essential to warm up the horse's muscles to prevent injury.
- Finish with a proper cool-down. This will allow the horse to lengthen its frame and release tension from the training session.
- Use positive reinforcement by praising the horse when it does well but do not punish or get frustrated when it does not. Remember, it might not be able to achieve what you are asking of it because of body restrictions, such as those relating to its conformation or pain.
- Gradually increase the intensity of training; this will help the horse to adapt to new exercises, in its body and mind.
- Ensure the tack is bespoke and the correct fit and check it monthly.
- Paying attention to the horse's body language can

help to identify any signs of discomfort or injury. Stop the training and re-evaluate if the horse shows discomfort or pain.
- Providing rest and recovery time can help to prevent injury and allow the horse's muscles and joints to repair and strengthen.
- Regularly evaluate the horse's fitness level and adapt the training accordingly: this can be performed by taking its vital signs, as noted in Chapter 1.

Consult a professional, especially if you are new to training horses, to help create a safe and effective training programme. Only use those with goals like yours, and you agree with their training methods. Do not think twice about changing a professional if they are not the right fit. Working with the wrong person can be very costly in the long run for you and your horse.

Positive responses from the horse include:

- Increased willingness to perform specific tasks or manoeuvres with better coordination and balance.
- Improved overall fitness and stamina.
- Greater confidence and trust in the rider.
- Increased muscle tone and definition.
- A more positive attitude towards training.
- An improved relationship and bonding.

Problem Solving

When the horse is trained incorrectly, there can be several negative consequences. It is not pleasant to watch a horse trained incorrectly; often, pain can be seen in the horse's face when it is struggling to move. Negative responses from the horse will tell you something is wrong and you need to investigate, such as:

- Grimacing when the horse is approached with its tack.
- Resistance to performing specific tasks or manoeuvres.
- Increased anxiety or stress levels.
- Aggression or other behavioural issues.
- Injury occurrences.
- Signs of lameness.

BODY SYSTEMS IN RESPONSE TO TRAINING

Exercise physiology is the study of how exercise affects the various systems of the body, including the cardiovascular, respiratory, neurological, muscular and skeletal systems. If a horse is not progressing as expected or showing negative responses to exercise, it could be due to the effects of exercise on one or more of these body systems, and further investigation is necessary.

Blood testing is a valuable tool for assessing a horse's fitness and overall health. It can help identify reasons for increased fatigue or the inability to cope with training, even when the horse seems fit. Blood tests can also screen for underlying infectious or metabolic diseases, such as viral infections or anaemia, which can affect the horse's performance.

Cardiovascular issues can lead to poor exercise performance in horses. Heart murmurs – caused by valve leakage and possible heart enlargement – can impair the heart's efficiency and compromise the circulation of oxygenated blood, resulting in rapid fatigue. Veterinarians use initial assessments with a stethoscope and may conduct additional diagnostic measures such as an ECG or ultrasound scan to determine the underlying cause.

Respiratory problems can also contribute to poor performance. Lower airway inflammation or laryngeal paralysis can cause heavy breathing, coughing or a whistling noise during exercise. Lung sounds are assessed with a stethoscope, and further diagnosis may involve endoscopy or tracheal wash. Restricting a horse's head position during exercise should be avoided as it can hinder airflow.

Metabolic conditions should be considered when addressing poor performance. Conditions such as Cushing's disease or low-grade liver disease can result in lacklustre or easily fatigued horses. Blood testing is helpful in confirming the diagnosis of these conditions.

Gastric ulceration, both in the stomach and hindgut, can significantly affect a horse's performance due to the pain it causes. Symptoms may include teeth grinding, tail swishing, headshaking and sensitivity of the region on palpation.

Musculoskeletal concerns should be thoroughly investigated. Stiffness or aversion to exercise without an apparent cause could indicate azoturia (tying up). Blood testing can help rule out other potential causes, such as storage myopathy, which affects the muscles' utilisation of nutrients.

★ TOP TIP

If the horse shows signs of lameness, it can refer to any difficulty or pain it experiences while moving. Common causes of lameness that you should consider are osteoarthritis due mainly to wear and tear; suspensory ligament, navicular bone; an infection that causes the horse to lose its balance (ataxia) and their ability to walk normally; laminitis that can be caused by grain consumption, hormones and obesity, poor nutrition resulting in hoof cracks; injuries such as bruised or punctured soles and abscesses that go undetected; conformation weaknesses; poorly fitting tack; rider asymmetry – as such, the horse incorrectly uses its body and this can manifest as lameness.

A proper diagnosis of lameness is essential to determine the underlying cause, develop an appropriate treatment plan and restructure the training plan. If the horse presents with lameness, the exercises and training plan should cease.

YOUR APPROACH TO TRAINING

Horse owners have different approaches because each person has their unique philosophy, beliefs and methods. Some people may prefer a more traditional approach, using techniques that have been used for centuries, such as classical dressage. Others may prefer a more modern approach, using techniques such as straightness training, at liberty, natural horsemanship, or positive reinforcement. People's experiences, backgrounds, and training can also influence their approach to training horses. For example, some people may have a background in a specific discipline, such as show jumping or eventing, while others may have an experience in therapy or rehabilitation. People may also have different goals for their horses, such as competition or recreation, which can also influence their approach to training.

As horses are individuals with unique personalities and characteristics, just like people, they have different learning styles and respond differently to training methods. Therefore, what works well for one horse may not work well for another. This means that people need to adjust their approach according to the individual horse's needs and characteristics.

It is more beneficial if the horse is trained naturally. Hence, the horse develops its shape and strength by correctly using its body without force or using gadgets or training aids that lock the horse's body into an unnatural shape, which is detrimental in the long term. It brings false muscle development, often done for a 'quick fix' to make the horse look good. Such horses might look attractive to a novice eye, but they will be sore and become injured over time. A trained eye with a therapy and rehabilitation background can look beyond this image and see lines of tension and unequal muscle development in the horse and how it compensates for this in its movement.

In practice, this means that every horse will move differently; some will be able to engage their hindquarters more efficiently and work in a nice frame, whilst others will need much more training, including strengthening other body parts that help with collection. It is the role of the owner to establish, early on, the capabilities of their horse and how they can train it to be the best it can be, and when errors occur in the horse's ridden frame, change what they are doing because it is not working for the horse – it will only result in injury. This takes time and patience: there are no 'quick fixes' when training horses.

AVOIDING PEER PRESSURE

This is very important when training your horse; you are responsible, no one else, and whilst some people may have good intentions, their advice might differ from what is needed. There are several ways to avoid peer pressure when training a horse:

- **Stay informed** – keep yourself updated about the latest training techniques and methods and research in equine behaviour, training and manual therapy. This will help you make informed decisions about your training programme rather than relying on others.
- **Trust your instincts** – you know your horse best and what works for it, so do not let other people's opinions or methods influence your training.
- **Evaluate the training outcome** – if the training is not producing positive results, it may be necessary to change the training programme.
- **Be open-minded** – try new methods and techniques, but also be willing to discard those that do not work for you and your horse.
- **Seek a mentor** with experience and knowledge in the area you are interested in who can provide guidance and support; this may be very different to what another person requires.
- **Seek compliance from the horse** – if the horse is uncomfortable with a particular method or technique, ensure you listen and take notice of what the horse is trying to convey; it is essential to stop and reassess.
- **Avoid pressure groups** that push a specific method or technique. Remember that every horse is different, and what works for one may not work for another.
- **Avoid social media** that does not offer expert advice; many equine groups offer conflicting and harmful advice because they are not always supported or underpinned by professional knowledge and experience.

Riding Styles and Exercise Choice

Ensure when riding in a particular style, it is done so correctly through the correct exercise choice, correct rider aids and responses from the horse, indicating that it understands and that its body can accomplish. The basis of most exercise starts with riding the horse on the bit, and it is the rider's responsibility to be able to encourage the horse to do this correctly. In practice, we see very few horses that are truly ridden on the bit, which is why we see so many musculoskeletal problems because the horse struggles to move its body and complete the tasks asked of it.

There are different opinions and perspectives on what constitutes acceptable riding styles in the equine world. Many musculoskeletal therapists find certain styles unacceptable because of the damage they inflict on the horse's body. Some equestrian judges may prioritise certain traditional riding styles and techniques, while others may emphasise modern, progressive methods that prioritise the horse's wellbeing. Having differing views across the equine industry is not uncommon on what is acceptable or cruel. For example, some professionals may consider certain training techniques, such as the use of harsh bits or excessive force, to be cruel and harmful to the horse. Others may view these techniques as necessary for achieving certain results in competition.

It is important to approach the sharing of information respectfully and educationally. Providing information to help riders reconsider their practices can contribute to promoting the wellbeing and welfare of horses. In the following sections, I include images and make comments that are not intended to criticise, I focus on facts, research, and make constructive suggestions in an attempt to provide you with informative and beneficial advice to help your horses to be pain-free.

ON THE BIT

Riding a horse 'on the bit' refers to a riding style in which the horse is in a state of balance and carrying the rider's weight through its hindquarters and allowing the horse to be responsive to the rider's aids. The horse's head and neck are naturally elevated, with the poll usually as the highest point. This is a good basis for all training but is not always easy to achieve. Being 'on the bit' makes the ride more comfortable for the horse and rider.

It is possible that a horse may be able to engage its hindquarters but still be 'leaning on the bit', which is a very common sight and is not one whereby the horse responds correctly to the rider's aids; it is therefore not truly 'on the bit'. This causes tension in the hindquarter and back muscles. It is also possible that a horse may be 'on the bit' but not adequately engaged in the hindquarters; in this case, the rider should work on developing the horse's hindquarters, impulsion and balance.

Helping a Horse to Work 'On the Bit'

The process can vary depending on the horse's individual needs and experience, but generally, it involves the following steps:

- Start with basic exercises to develop the horse's strength, flexibility and balance. This can include

> ★ **TOP TIP**
>
> Ultimately, it is up to individual horse owners, riders, trainers and judges to make ethical and responsible choices regarding the welfare of horses. I firmly believe it is important to prioritise the horse's health and wellbeing above winning competitions or conforming to certain traditional standards. By working together and promoting responsible horsemanship, we can create a more compassionate and sustainable equine industry. Producing a book about manual therapy and everything that underpins it is a good start, in my opinion!

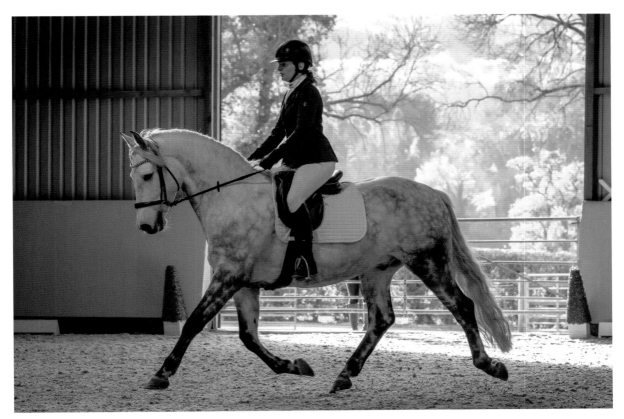

The horse is 'on the bit', displaying engaged hindquarters with stepping under hind limbs and an engaged core lifting the back and freeing the shoulders, enabling a full forelimb range of motion. The head and neck exhibit good posture as the horse works uphill, while pricked ears and soft eyes indicate contentment.

groundwork – such as lunging and long-lining – and some ridden work, such as transitions, pole work and bending exercises.

- Gradually introduce the horse to the bit and the rider's aids, ensuring the horse is comfortable and relaxed. Using a mild bit is an advantage.
- Develop the horse's forward movement and impulsion, encouraging the horse to move forward into the bit.
- As the horse becomes more responsive, work on refining the horse's balance and engagement by asking for exercises such as half-halts in a walk to trot, then trot to canter and, later on, more collection work.
- Always be consistent in your training and be patient. It can take time for a horse to understand and accept the bit correctly. It is important to note that

this process should always be done with the horse's wellbeing in mind, avoiding any form of harshness or using training aids to 'force' the horse, as this is not truly 'on the bit'. A good rider should be able to get the horse 'on the bit' with a good balance and with a relaxed state of mind.

ABOVE THE BIT

Riding a horse 'above the bit' can lead to the horse being pulled off balance and causing discomfort. Therefore, it is considered a less desirable riding style and can signify poor training or riding technique. Often unfit or young horses work 'above the bit', as their musculature, balance and posture mean they are not strong enough to work 'on the bit'; if this is the case, they need pre-training but never force.

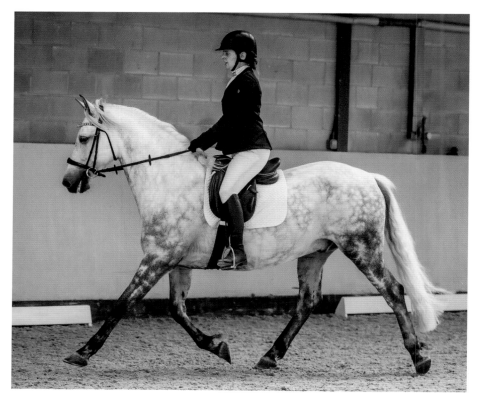

The horse is demonstrating 'above the bit', with a non-vertical head position, but still displaying forward movement. The shoulder is light, forelimbs extend well, while the hindquarters lack engagement, limiting hindlimb range and tracking up. The back is moderately hollowed, and the core is partially engaged.

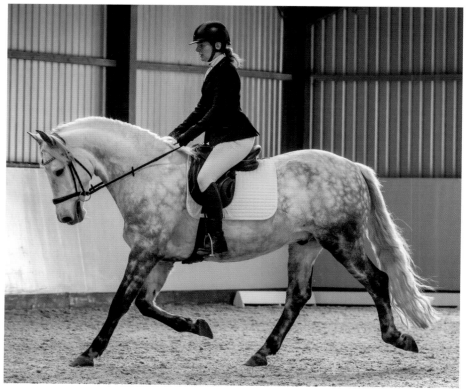

The horse is demonstrating 'behind the bit', lacking hindquarter engagement and hindlimb range, inhibiting tracking up. The back is hollowed, the core partially engaged and the shoulders restricted due to being on the forehand, resulting in limited forelimb movement and a downhill posture. The horse appears content and relaxed, but a limitation in the throat latch area may impact breathing.

BEHIND THE BIT

Riding a horse 'behind the bit' refers to a riding style in which the horse is not engaged correctly and is not carrying itself in a balanced way. The horse may be 'leaning on the bit', meaning it is not properly accepting the rider's aids. This can result in a lack of responsiveness and impulsion, making it difficult for the rider to maintain correct balance, control and communication with the horse. It can also cause discomfort or pain for the horse. This is also considered a less desirable riding style and can be a sign of poor training or riding technique.

Often young or unfit horses work 'behind the bit' as they are unlikely to have strong enough musculature to work 'on the bit', and 'behind the bit' is more manageable for it, but the horse then ends up 'on the forehand', which is not good for balance.

HYPERFLEXION

This is where the horse is overbent and held in an unnatural frame. This is considered a harmful and painful riding style that puts pressure on the horse's spine; it restricts the forelimbs and shoulders so the horse cannot lift the shoulder and work in an uphill movement. This posture can also put excess pressure on the lower part of the neck's cervical vertebrae and the poll. All horses ridden in this style show indicators of pain in their face and have tension in their musculoskeletal system.

Hyperflexion in a Dressage Horse

Although many equestrians, including dressage enthusiasts, might believe the following image is attractive, it is not to those of us that work in therapy and rehabilitation with horses; this horse is overbent to the degree that the horse will have a great deal of tension in its body.

Research has shown that horses regularly ridden in this frame have overstretched vertebrae; some were found to have fractures in the vertebrae due to this unnatural positioning and muscular development of the neck. The spine is subjected to abnormal move-

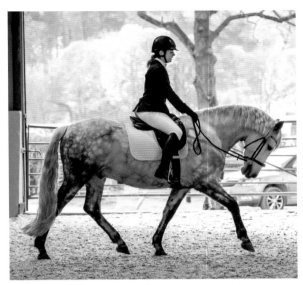

The horse demonstrates 'hyperflexion' with a restricted poll, throat and neck. This limits the full extension of the forelimbs and restricts shoulder movement. It lacks engagement of hindquarters and core, resulting in a hollowed back.

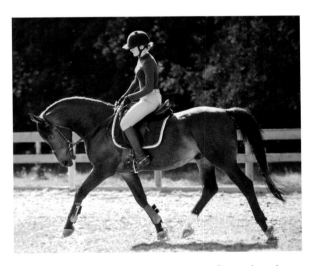

The horse demonstrates severe 'hyperflexion', with excessive neck bending, restricting shoulder and forelimb movement, and straining the poll, neck vertebrae and muscles. This hinders the core and hindquarters engagement, causing a hollowed back. The horse is on the forehand, indicating weight distribution towards the front legs. It displays a pained expression with an open mouth and a staring eye. This forced frame is damaging and could lead to long-term soundness issues despite the horse's athleticism.

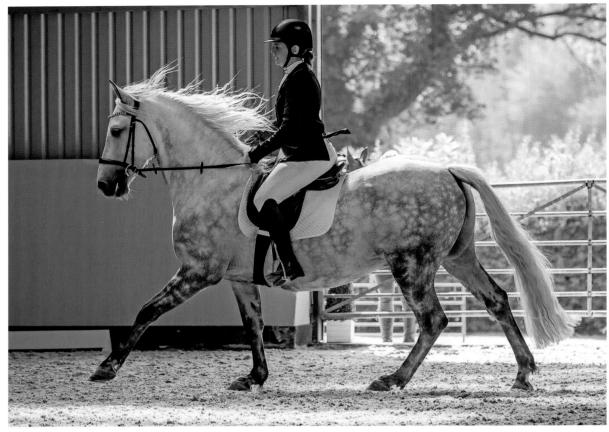

The horse is demonstrating a 'downwardly flexed topline' with a high head and neck position and hollow back, which means its hindquarters are not engaged and are placed behind the horse. The forelimb can be seen to be extending forward also. Hence this frame is also referred to as being ridden in 'extension'. The horse's face looks happy, with ears forward, but there is some foam around the bit, suggesting some tension in the mouth.

ment, which can affect the spinal cord. This is a good example of an industry accepting standards that are not beneficial for the horse.

DOWNWARDLY FLEXED TOPLINE 'EXTENSION'

Downwardly flexed topline is a less desirable style of riding. This means that the core muscles are not engaged, and the muscles along the top of the horse's neck, back and hindquarters are contracted, causing the horse's back to be hollow. In this position, the horse's weight is shifted to its forehand, and its hindquarters are less engaged, resulting in decreased impulsion and power. The horse's breathing can also

be affected, since the muscles used for respiration are connected to the topline, which can restrict the horse's ability to take full breaths, limiting its oxygen intake and stamina.

Eventers and show jumping horses are often seen moving in a 'downwardly flexed topline' with their head high and hollow back because it is a natural posture for them to take when jumping. This posture allows the horse to see and judge the distance to the jump better and to take off at the right spot. Additionally, this posture allows them to land more comfortably by absorbing the impact of the landing with their front legs while their hindquarters remain elevated and ready for the next stride. However, it is important to note that this posture should only be used during jumping and not during other phases of training or riding, as it can cause long-term damage to the horse's spine and muscles if used excessively. It can also be referred to as the horse moving in 'extension', because of the extended limb positioning.

UPWARDLY FLEXED TOPLINE 'COLLECTION' WITH HIGH HEAD

An upwardly flexed topline is more beneficial. This means that the core muscles are engaged whilst the muscles along the top of the horse's neck, back and hindquarters are relaxed and elongated, causing the horse's back to be rounded and its head and neck to be raised. In this position, the horse's weight is shifted towards its hindquarters and its hind legs are more engaged, resulting in increased impulsion and power. The horse's breathing can also be improved, since the muscles used for respiration can function more effectively in this position, allowing for better oxygen intake and stamina.

This riding style is often seen in dressage, in which the horse is asked to perform a variety of precise movements, such as lateral work and collected canter. The rider's position and the horse's way of going should be balanced and harmonious to achieve the 'upwardly flexed topline' or 'collection'. It is considered one of the higher levels of training. It is typically only achievable after a horse has progressed through several stages of training and developed the necessary

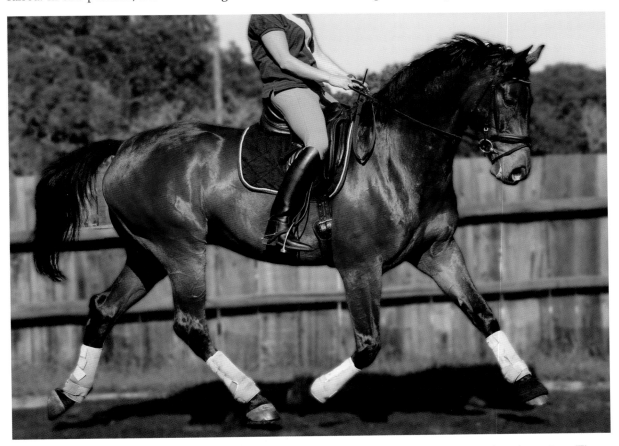

This horse is being ridden in an 'upwardly flexed topline' or 'collection' with an elevated neck carriage. The horse's core and hindquarters are engaged and balanced, with a lifted and rounded back that supports the rider. The horse is moving in an uphill frame with a fluid gait, indicating good tracking up. Tension is evident in the horse's face, and foam around the mouth suggests some discomfort in this position, or overworking.

muscle strength and flexibility, which will be covered in further sections of this chapter. This is achieved mainly through the rider's aids. The horse is not kept in place by the hands or training aids; the hands are only used to recycle the energy produced by the rider's seat and legs. The collected appearance results from the activity of the horse's hindquarters. The test is if the rider lets go of both reins; the horse should stay in collection for several strides.

UPWARDLY FLEXED TOPLINE 'COLLECTION' WITH LOW HEAD CARRIAGE

It is possible to ride a horse in 'collection' without a high head carriage, which can be a more comfortable and sustainable posture for the horse. However, achieving this requires proper training and strength in the horse and a proficient rider who can guide the horse into this frame.

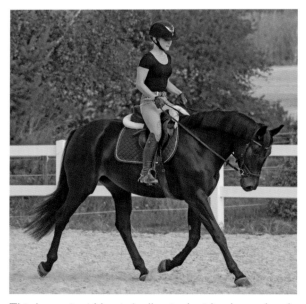

This horse is ridden in 'collection' with a lower head and neck carriage but is still balanced. The horse is tracking up, engaging its core, lifting and rounding its back. The head and neck are in a lower frame, but the shoulder has a good range of motion, and the forelimbs are not restricted. There are no signs of discomfort in the horse's expression.

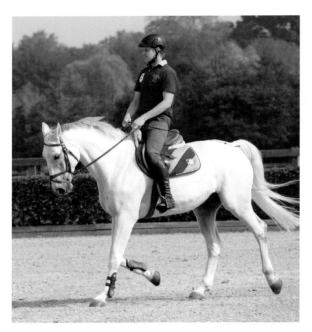

This horse is ridden 'on the forehand' with its nose pointing towards the front feet. The forelimb range of motion is restricted, and the hindquarters are not engaged to push forward and allow the horse to lift at the front end. It is not balanced. Some horses are ridden with the nose pointing more acutely towards their front feet than in the image, which is very unbalancing.

ON THE FOREHAND

Riding a horse 'on the forehand' means that most of the horse's weight is carried on its front legs. This results in the horse being heavy on the forehand, with its hindquarters trailing behind and not engaged in the movement.

When a horse is ridden on the forehand, it can make it difficult for the horse to maintain balance and impulsion, and it can also put additional strain on the horse's front legs. It is generally considered an undesirable way of riding a horse and can be corrected through proper training and riding techniques.

LONG AND LOW

Riding a horse 'long and low' refers to a style of riding and training that emphasises the horse being ridden in a long, low frame with a relaxed and supple top line.

The horse is asked to stretch out and work in a low, extended frame, with the head and neck held low and the back rounded. This style of riding is often used in the training of dressage horses, as it helps to promote suppleness, flexibility and balance in the horse. It also encourages the horse to engage its hindquarters and use its back more effectively.

The horse is worked in a relatively low frame, with little contact on the bit. The focus is maintaining a steady rhythm, forward movement and a relaxed, swinging back. This training helps improve the horse's fitness and musculature, making them stronger and more capable of performing advanced movements. It also helps to improve their posture and carriage, improving their overall appearance. This is not a novice style of riding; it takes time to achieve true 'long and low', as the horse must be strong enough and balanced beforehand.

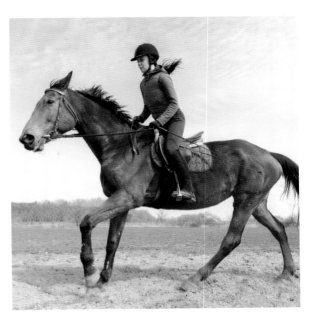

This horse lacks overall condition and has muscle weakness throughout its body; it is weak and unbalanced. The lack of gluteal muscling and hamstring overdevelopment attempts to support a weak pelvis. If this horse is not strengthened and conditioned with gradual, proper training, starting with rest, a nutrition review, and then pre-training, it will inevitably injure and likely break down. It would be challenging to fit a saddle to this horse.

WEAK AND UNBALANCED

A weak, unbalanced horse lacks physical strength, energy and vitality due to many factors, such as poor or incorrect nutrition, illness, lack of correct training and undiagnosed conditions, such as gastric or hindgut ulcers and worm burden. Some horses have proper nutrition, with no disease present but still need to be stronger and more balanced with the correct training.

An unbalanced horse has an uneven distribution of weight and muscles with atrophy present; it would not be able to perform certain tasks, such as being ridden 'on the bit' or 'in collection' because it is too weak. Unbalanced horses are prone to injury and have difficulty moving comfortably or efficiently. As well as the proper training, they also require specific management.

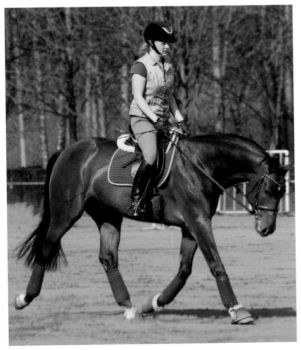

This horse is ridden in a 'long and low' frame with a soft mouth and tracking up well. Its back is lifting, and core engaged, but it could be slightly more forward going with more hindquarter engagement. The gait looks fluid, the muscles look supple, and there is no evidence of tension.

WARM-UP AND COOL-DOWN

The process of warming up a horse before exercise is different from the concept of riding 'long and low'. The objective of the 'warm-up' is to prepare the horse's muscles and body for more intensive work, including increasing the heart rate and breathing, loosening the joints and muscles and improving overall flexibility and range of motion. Conversely, the 'cool-down' aims to help the horse's body return to a state of rest and recovery after exercise by reducing the heart rate and breathing, preventing the build-up of lactic acid in the muscles, and alleviating muscle fatigue.

To accomplish these goals, the horse should be ridden in a calm, relaxed manner throughout the warm-up and cool-down periods, focusing on progressively increasing or decreasing the horse's heart rate and breathing and enhancing the horse's flexibility and range of motion. Starting and ending with a loose rein to allow the horse to stretch is essential.

During the warm-up, the rider should begin with a few minutes of walking on a loose rein, allowing the horse to become comfortable with the bit and rider

aids. The rider can then gradually increase the pace to a trot and canter, using large circles and direction changes to loosen the horse's joints and muscles. As the horse's body warms up, the rider can incorporate more complex movements, such as leg yields, shoulder-in and other lateral exercises, if the horse is ready.

During the cool-down, the rider should gradually decrease the pace, starting with a canter and then transitioning to a trot and walk. The rider should focus on stretching and flexing the horse's muscles and joints, performing large circles and serpentines at the walk. As the horse's body cools down, the rider should allow some standing time and let the horse stretch its head and neck towards the ground.

Throughout the warm-up and cool-down, the rider should monitor the horse's breathing and heart rate, adjusting the intensity of the exercises as necessary. The rider should also pay attention to the horse's response and adjust the pace or movements if the horse seems fatigued or uncomfortable. Warming up and cooling down should be done progressively to help the horse adjust to the new demands placed on its body.

The duration of both warm-up and cool-down should be relative to the amount and intensity of the work the horse will be doing. In a thirty-minute schooling session, at least ten minutes should be spent in the warm-up, followed by ten minutes of varied schooling with rest periods and at least ten minutes in cool-down. Research suggests that dividing the horse's schooling work in this way into thirds is very beneficial. Neglecting warm-up, proper training and cool-down can result in many horses having muscle problems and requiring professional musculoskeletal therapy, making it crucial to adhere to these principles.

You must ensure that if you have booked a riding lesson with your horse and your instructor requires you to work during the session with a minimum warm-up and cool-down, you allocate sufficient time to do this before and after the lesson.

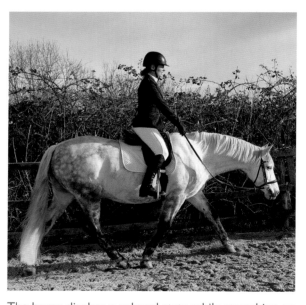

The horse displays a relaxed state while stretching on a loose rein, and his breathing can regulate following a schooling session. The rider is not dictating the horse's shape.

Facial Expressions Indicating the Presence of Pain

This is a good opportunity to introduce the Grimace Scale, a tool used to assess pain in horses, which was developed as part of a study by a group of researchers led by Emanuela Dalla Costa, published online in 2014. The scale utilises specific facial expressions or 'grimaces' associated with pain, which are scored based on the presence and intensity of certain facial features, such as ear position, eye shape, nostril shape, face tension, lip retraction and mouth opening. The scale has since been widely adopted as an effective way to evaluate pain in horses, both in clinical settings and in research studies. Later, Sue Dyson *et al* conducted a study published in 2017 that validated the horse grimace scale as a reliable method for assessing pain in ridden horses, indicating its usefulness as a tool for monitoring equine welfare.

I strongly advise adopting this principle with your horses, whether ridden or not. In my work, I rely on this to determine the pain levels of the horses; some are retired, and some compete, but whatever their situation, it does provide a good indicator of what the horse might be experiencing. I am not suggesting that this will be accurate in every case, but certainly I have found a correlation after observing facial expressions and then conducting palpation that pain is likely to be present. Pain negatively affects a horse's wellbeing and performance; thus, a horse in pain is not acceptable. Pain management in horses involves addressing other factors such as the riding style, tack and other influences that may contribute to pain and injury, leading to negative impacts on the horse's physical and mental health.

Regarding salivation, it is worth noting that, in my experience, it is not necessarily a relaxation response. In many instances, it is a stressor resulting from the horse working too hard or being uncomfortable in its mouth, with its breathing affected, leading to salivation. Salivation is often observed in horses working intensely 'on the bit' or in 'hyperflexion'.

Facial expressions in studies, that were scientifically deemed to indicate the presence of pain, include:

★ TOP TIP

As a horse owner, it is essential to ensure your horse's wellbeing. Pain is a significant factor that can negatively impact your horse's physical and mental health. To incorporate facial expressions as a valuable welfare tool for your own horses, I recommend that you first familiarise yourself with the expressions and features to assess, such as ear position, eye shape, nostril shape, face tension, lip retraction and mouth opening, revealing the teeth and the tongue. Then regularly, observe your horse's face, looking for signs of discomfort or pain in ridden and non-ridden work. Score your horse's facial expressions based on the indicators provided to determine if they are experiencing no pain, mild to moderate pain, or severe pain.

This will help you to better assess and manage your horse and ensure it is as comfortable and healthy as it can be. Remember that appropriate pain management, including monitoring your horse's tack and riding style, its feet and teeth and its muscle health, are essential to maintaining their well-being.

A NORMAL RESPONSE

The horse's head is relaxed and working on the bit, its ears are facing forward, its eye is open and a rounded shape with no orbital tension, its nostrils are relaxed, and its mouth is closed and relaxed.

MILD TO MODERATE PAIN INDICATORS

The head might be twisted to one side, below the bit or above the bit, one ear might face to the side and one to the back. The eye is open and almond shape, or the eye is half closed. The mouth is slightly separated, but no teeth are showing, or the mouth is open slightly, and teeth and tongue can be seen.

SEVERE PAIN INDICATORS

The head can be below the bit or above the bit, with both ears facing back. The eye is almost closed and can show the white (sclera) or an intense stare or worried look, and tension in the orbital muscles around the eye. There is a wrinkle between the nostrils or an angular profile of the nostrils rather than a rounded one. The mouth can be open wide, teeth can be seen and possibly the tongue. The bit might be pulled to the side.

In the following images, I will classify the pain levels as I observe them following the research guidelines. Nevertheless, it is crucial to mention that further evaluation and palpation, which I will discuss in Chapter 6, can provide a more accurate indication of the pain category. However, using the images as a starting point can be extremely beneficial and very useful to compare with your own horses.

Choosing an ethical and kinder way to ride your horse is not only the responsible thing to do for its welfare, but it also demonstrates a commitment to creating a more compassionate and sustainable equine industry. By prioritising a horse's wellbeing above traditional methods, riders can build a stronger bond with their equine partners and set an example for others to follow. Combined with the horse receiving regular manual therapy during all stages of its training, you support it the best way you can. As the exercises change and progress, the horse will be challenged in its body and might become sore in certain muscle groups, which you can promptly address.

Improving circulation during exercise, relieving muscle tension, and improving range of motion through manual therapy, benefits the horse's performance and overall wellbeing during any training programme. Plan your pre-competition massage before the event, post-competition afterwards and a regular maintenance massage routine. You will see a difference in your horse. However, if you feel that your horse is presenting with something beyond your manual therapy skills, then you can enlist a trained professional musculoskeletal therapist to help.

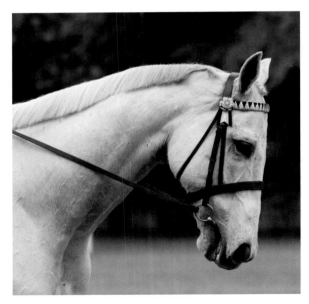

Mild to moderate pain category as the eye shows signs of orbital tension and is partially closed. The horse's mouth is open, revealing its tongue. The ears are not facing forward, and the nostrils appear angular instead of rounded, indicating that the horse may even fall under the severe pain category.

Mild to moderate pain category as the eye shows some orbital tension, the ears are not facing forward, the nostrils have an angular profile instead of being rounded, and there is tension in the mouth. The horse's mouth is open, and the tongue and teeth are visible.

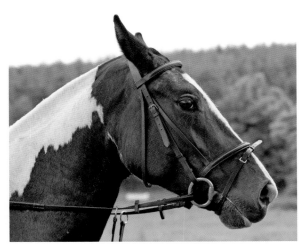

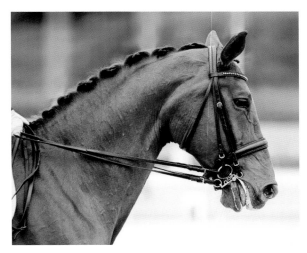

Mild to moderate category as the horse's ears are back, and the eye appears tense. Additionally, the flash noseband is tied too tightly, causing additional pressure and pain on the facial nerves. The horse's head is above the bit at an angle of more than 30 per cent, which could indicate the severe pain category.

Severe pain category. The ears are not facing forward, there is orbital tension in the horse's eye. The horse is more than 30 per cent above the bit, which indicates excessive pressure on the tongue, causing the mouth to be open, and the tongue to be visible with foam present. In addition, there is nostril tension with an angular profile, which is an additional sign of severe pain.

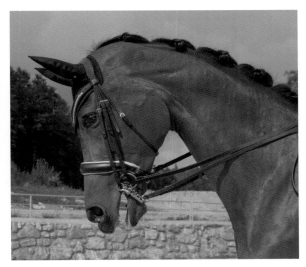

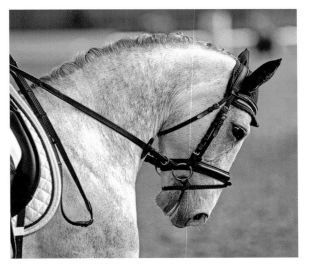

Severe pain category. Although the ears are facing forward, the horse's eye shows signs of tension with a fixed stare. The nostrils appear wide, and the skin inside looks red, indicating pressure. There is a great deal of strain in the horse's mouth, which is open wide, and the tongue appears under extreme pressure. Although the horse's head is placed vertically, there is visible tension in the throat area, indicating the horse's breathing may be affected.

Severe pain category. The ears are not facing forward, there is intense tension in the horse's eye. The horse is more than 30 per cent behind the bit, which indicates excessive pressure on the mouth, causing tension and opening of the mouth despite a clamped flash noseband. The nostrils have an angular profile, indicating increased pressure and pain. The horse also shows signs of strain in breathing, possibly due to the neck position.

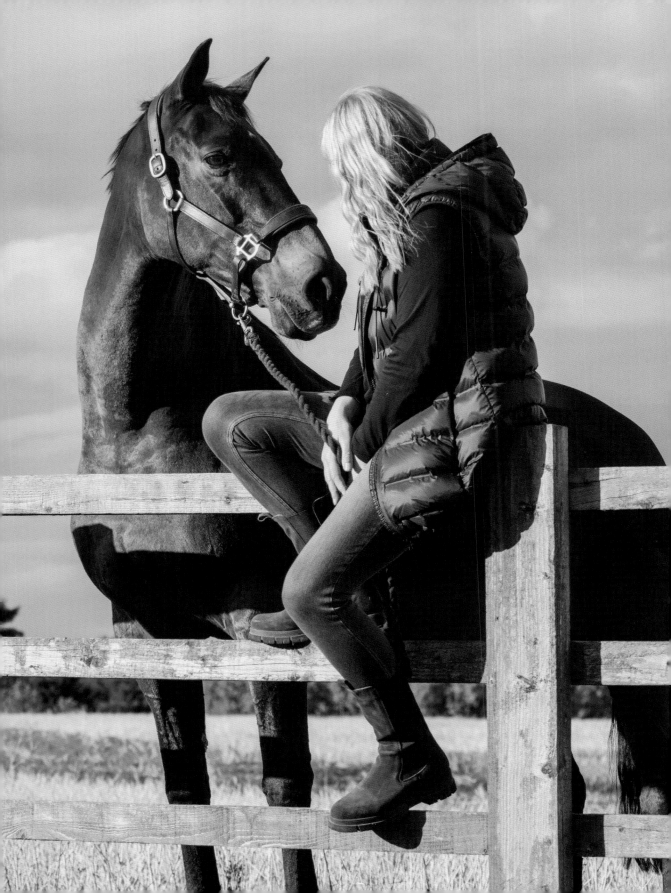

CHAPTER 5

Knowledge and Preparation

Scope of Training and Working Within the Law

Horse owners can perform any manual therapy on their horses, but it is against the law to perform it on another person's horse if you have not been formally trained as a therapist and are not fully insured. When looking for a professional to attend to your horse, ensure they have completed a recognised, accredited training course, which involves theory and clinical hours working with horses. I recommend a level three course at the minimum, but a level five offers an excellent standard.

Some inadequate training providers qualify people in less than a week, which harms the industry and horses' health. No one can adequately qualify in this timescale; most reputable courses are no less than one-year duration with lots of studying, comprising assignments and case studies so that the student can progress as a therapist through continual assessment and expert feedback from experienced assessors and instructors. Once qualified, they should be fully insured (professional indemnity and public liability) and be committed to career-long learning, which is continual professional development training (CPD).

An appropriately qualified person will work within the legal framework and observe the relevant legislation of their country of operation, which in the UK is the Veter- inary Surgery (Exemptions) Order 2015. They may also become members of a professional organisation within their country of operation, and such memberships reflect legal, professional and ethical requirements that members must adhere to in their conduct and clinical practice when working with horses.

No one should ever work outside their scope of practice, whether they are a horse owner or a professional. Everyone must understand their limitations; otherwise, what they do to a horse might be damaging and beyond repair.

Manual Therapy Terminology

Manual therapy will influence the entire musculoskeletal system of your horse; it is a more general term that encompasses various techniques used to treat musculoskeletal problems in horses. Whilst the terminology to describe the therapy and its techniques may differ, the principles behind them are the same: manual therapy, massage therapy, physiotherapy, bodywork and so on, all aim to improve the horse's well-being; I referred to this briefly at the beginning of Chapter 2.

I feel it is important to compare equine manual therapy to that available for people. At a spa, a therapist may provide a general relaxation massage, applying the same techniques from head to toe for every client; we might adopt this approach when offering a horse a 'maintenance massage'. On the other hand, a specialist trained in various massage styles would address the specific condition of the client, such as neck or back pain, which is our approach with horses during a 'remedial massage'. Additionally, athletes may receive an authentic sports massage before and after competing to prepare their muscles for the extra workload and minimise the risk of injury and to help them recover afterwards; we would offer this to a horse as a 'sports massage' before and after competing.

Manual therapy, including massage and other therapeutic techniques, can provide various benefits depending on their application. It is essential to determine what is optimal for your horse, considering its physical and psychological requirements, such as its current health status, transition from one career to another, workload demands, level of competition and whether the horse is recovering from an injury.

With horses, the ambient temperature is also essential when deciding on manual therapy and the techniques of choice. For example, suppose you intend to warm the tissues before a competition by performing a sports massage (pre-competition), which is perfectly acceptable, but if it is a hot day, then you do not want to warm the tissues too much and divert blood, oxygen and nutrients away from the vital organs and bodily systems, so you would perform less of the warming techniques and focus on those that would help release muscle fibres more. Conversely, on a colder day, your focus could be more on warming the tissues to increase circulation.

This book provides a partial range of techniques for horse owners because a full range, used professionally, should only be performed after extensive training underpinned with comprehensive anatomy and physiology knowledge. It is aimed at owners who want to gain more understanding by learning how to assess their horses and apply manual therapy for maximum benefit.

I have intentionally provided several categories of manual therapy that can be effectively translated and applied to your horse from reading this book. I repeat that complex techniques, mobilisations, manipulations or stretching of horses should only be used with extensive professional training; if performed without the necessary training, they can be harmful.

The various categories that make up 'manual therapy' can be applied alone or combined with other treatment modalities, such as correct supportive exercise, electrotherapy, hydrotherapy, medication and more, to enhance the overall health and wellbeing of the horse.

Categories of Manual Therapy

MYOFASCIAL RELEASE

Myofascial release is a manual therapy I introduced into my training company in 2010 whilst still in its infancy in human treatment. It proved to be gentle yet effective, and was particularly well-received by horses. Scientific studies conducted later on have validated the benefits of myofascial release, confirming what I had already discovered and taught years ago, indicating we were ahead of our time.

The fascial system can face challenges due to various factors, such as trauma, postural changes, the influence of tack or riders and incorrect training methods. Inflammation resulting from injuries, inadequate recovery, lack of rest days and excessive demands on the horse can also affect the fascia. Additionally, inactivity caused by confinement or limited turnout can impact fascial health. These factors can lead to restrictions and adhesions in the fascia, which can exert abnormal pressure on the horse's nerves, muscles, bones and organs. Therefore, it is crucial for horses to have regular movement and turnout to maintain their wellbeing.

Myofascial release focuses on addressing specific areas of the body with fascial restrictions, pain and abnormal movements, thereby promoting freer movement for the horse. Its primary benefits lie in improving blood circulation, nutrient and oxygen delivery and lymphatic flow. The fascia, being the largest sensory organ in the body, plays a significant role in the horse's nervous system. Releasing the fascia through myofascial release can have a positive impact on the horse's nervous system, often resulting in a reset-like response in the horse's brain. This can be observed through moments of staring, blinking and sometimes small jolting movements, eventually leading to complete relaxation.

TENSION POINT RELEASE (TPR)

I founded TPR for horses after witnessing how many horses could not tolerate traditional forms of human touch, mostly due to their emotional tension, which manifested as physical tension. Through extensive research and experimentation after working with Group One racehorses in Europe, China, Hong Kong, Singapore and the United Arab Emirates, I discovered that gentle pressure on specific tension points throughout the horse's body could provide therapeutic benefits without causing discomfort or stress. This led me to develop tension point release to help horses receive the healing benefits of touch in a way that is comfortable and effective for them. These points can be found at specific body junctions, over muscle and bone. I must stipulate there that this is different to trigger point therapy and any similar therapies involving gentle touch.

Applying TPR to the correct tension point in the body can bring profound results. This is because TPR focuses on specific areas of the body, mainly at bone landmarks where we know tension to commonly sit in most horses due to their anatomy and what we do with them that brings challenges for their body parts. Horses are emotionally challenged in their daily existence, and TPR can work on that level also.

MASSAGE

Massage is a broad term and can include a variety of techniques aimed at compressing, kneading, rubbing and stretching muscles performed in long or short strokes with varying pressure. The different styles can create a variety of benefits, from relaxation to pain relief within a muscle. All manual therapy, including massage, works with various body systems, as highlighted in Chapter 2.

Massage is a practice founded on knowledge from ancient civilisations from China, Japan, India, Egypt, Greece and Rome. The terminology used in massage can be unclear as many French words describe a Swedish massage style. This highlights the various influences of civilisations practised today in human massage – many of which have been translated to horses effectively.

This chapter will provide succinct descriptions of the techniques I will demonstrate and overcomplicated terminology and explanations will be avoided. The aim is for you to have knowledge and understanding of the best techniques that will benefit your horse both physically and psychologically, which are performed to meet specific needs.

Deep tissue massage is a style of massage that focuses on the deeper layers of muscles and connective tissue; however, the pressure applied is often more intense than that generally used with horses and, as such, it can be very uncomfortable. A therapist working with a human patient would find a level that

★ TOP TIP

On occasions, I have visited horses that have received a deep tissue massage from another differently trained therapist, and the horse has been in pain because the deep tissue approach has bruised already vulnerable tissue and has caused inflammation because a bespoke approach was not adopted and a generic one used instead. Anyone offering manual therapy should, in my opinion, fully assess the horse first so they know which techniques to use. There are other more suitable techniques to use with horses; as such, deep tissue will not be taught in this book.

is effective and comfortable for the patient through their communication. However, I do not find deep tissue massage to be one that can be translated to the horse from human massage. I have found it to be of little or no benefit during my many years of experience.

The sub-categories of massage refer to the different approaches including sports massage (pre-competition and post-competition), maintenance and remedial.

Sports Massage (Pre-Competition and Post-Competition)

The term sports massage has been overused and often misused when relating to horses. Therefore, my explanation and use might differ from others in the industry; I would only use sports massage as terminology for pre-competition and post-competition massages with horses, not as a category of massage for muscle injury, pain or tension; I have other specific types for these scenarios.

Pre-Competition

Pre-competition sports massage is a targeted approach aimed at preparing equine athletes for strenuous activities, such as competitive events or intense training sessions. The goal is to realign and loosen muscle fibres, improve blood circulation, oxygen and nutrient supply, and overall prepare the horse's body for increased work while reducing the risk of sport-related tension and injuries.

Ideally, the massage should be performed within four hours before the competition, as the horse can still benefit from its effects during the event. If travelling to a competition, the massage can be done the evening before. Upon arrival at the destination, after the horse has settled and recovered from the journey, gentle techniques can be applied until the moment of riding. However, it is important to be mindful of certain limitations. Consider the ambient temperature and avoid overheating the horse through excessive massage, as it would place further demands on its body during competition. Additionally, travel can be demanding on the horse's musculoskeletal system, causing muscle fatigue and dehydration. The focus of pre-competition massage is to stimulate and warm the tissues, rather than fatigue them.

It is crucial to adapt the techniques based on each horse's individual needs and preferences. Vibratory techniques such as Tapotement should be avoided if the horse is anxious, as they can overstimulate certain individuals. Massage should always be individualised and tailored to the specific horse's requirements.

Techniques include:

- Effleurage
- Tapotement
- Shaking
- Myofascial release

Post-Competition

This type of massage is performed after any competitive event or strenuous schooling session or even a long hack. Its purpose is to speed up the healing process, allowing the horse to recover more quickly. Muscle soreness is minimised, as is swelling due to fluid accumulation in the tissues, such as lactic acid, which occurs after more strenuous exercise and can cause stiffness and pain for the horse. Horses competing are also performing repetitive movements. If there is an unknown underlying condition in the horse's body – for example, osteoarthritis of the hock – then this could result in pain in that region, which needs time to recover. It is also an excellent opportunity to perform a health and safety check on your horse to ascertain if it has encountered any injuries while competing or travelling.

The post-competition massage would be performed at least two hours after the competition when homeostasis is present, that is when the horse is rehydrated, no sweating is evident and its vital signs have returned to normal. If the horse has travelled after an event, the post-competition massage can be performed later that evening or the following morning, depending on the time of day it competes or when the strenuous work is undertaken.

After strenuous activity, the horse's muscles are vulnerable, and damage could occur if the horse is worked too quickly. For example, if the horse sustained a micro tear in a muscle whilst competing, if it is not massaged and rested for at least twenty-four hours but preferably forty-eight, and returns to regular activity almost immediately, the micro tear could develop as a more damaging tear. Therefore, manual therapy, rest and gentle walking are always recommended to allow the horse time to heal after competing. If a horse regularly competes, then including the post-competition massage into the horse's schedule can help the horse to feel better and return to work better equipped. The focus is to soothe tissues and help expel waste products to enhance recovery rates.

Techniques include:

- Effleurage
- Shaking
- Myofascial release

Maintenance Massage

A maintenance massage is a regularly scheduled massage for horses, regardless of any existing injuries, pain, tension or performance issues. It is a non-specific approach to check and monitor the horse's muscle condition and address any concerns before they develop into significant problems. Regular maintenance massages can help prevent the recurrence of historical issues, such as previous injuries, by providing ongoing manual therapy and adjusting training accordingly.

Some horse owners prefer to perform maintenance massages on a weekly or monthly basis, although there is no fixed schedule. The more frequently the massages are done, especially on a weekly basis, the better chance there is of detecting and preventing musculoskeletal issues early on. Additionally, certain treatment techniques can be incorporated into the maintenance massage to focus on specific body parts, similar to remedial massages.

Horses that work in flexion or with training aids can also benefit from maintenance massages to relieve muscle tension in various areas of the body. Young horses undergoing physical changes, career transitions such as racehorse to riding horse, or brood mares carrying foals can benefit from gentle maintenance massages as well. For horses with high-stress workloads, busy competition schedules, or anxiety, maintenance massages are a valuable addition to their training routine, helping alleviate accumulated muscle tension. Also, they are very beneficial with horses on box rest to help restore mobility and muscle tone.

Techniques include:

- Effleurage
- Compression
- Shaking
- Friction
- Myofascial release

Remedial Massage

Remedial massage is the most common category for a musculoskeletal therapist, focusing on recovery and rehabilitation. The horse's soft tissues are treated for a specific therapeutic effect rather than a general result. Such as, if the horse is not going well, there may be some muscle tension and soreness: the focus would be on specific known muscle injuries or a sore back from wearing an incorrectly fitting saddle. Using relevant techniques and pressures according to the horse's needs and responses enhances the healing process, helping repair the soft tissues and restoring functionality by adapting the tissues and the horse back to a healthy state.

Although the focus is similar, there are differences between the terms 'remedial' and 'rehabilitation' that you might hear. Remedial massage is a therapy that aims to treat the soft tissues that are damaged, tense, immobile and painful. Rehabilitation is restoring something that has been damaged to its former condition. Both meanings are very similar, but in a professional capacity, the term rehabilitation also includes the correct supportive exercise programme we recommend. The professional therapists I teach are highly trained in both, so they can address the entire horse with a targeted approach.

We would only advocate passive stretching to the horse during a remedial massage by a qualified therapist. This could be useful to help lengthen tissue that has been restricted during box rest or to help mobilise tissue around a specific healed injured site. I do, however, prefer to perform the myofascial release technique on scar tissue as opposed to stretching the horse, because it is gentle but very effective and does not involve a limb being repositioned as in a stretch, which could result in further damage.

To avoid inflicting any more damage to soft tissues, I recommend a gentle, non-invasive approach for horse owners that can bring excellent results when applied correctly.

Techniques include:

- Effleurage
- Compression
- Shaking
- Friction
- Myofascial release

MUSCLE INJURY SPECIFICS AND STRATEGIES FOR REPAIR

When a horse experiences a mild to moderate muscle injury, utilising appropriate manual therapy during the appropriate stage of healing can be greatly advantageous. However, identifying a muscle injury can be challenging unless it is apparent, such as when a horse overextends or incorrectly navigates an obstacle, potentially resulting in a micro muscle tear. Palpating the horse to determine tenderness in the affected region is necessary to confirm such an injury. In the case of severe muscle injury, such as those resulting from a significant fall, it is imperative to seek veterinary support, since other bodily damage may have occurred.

Inflammatory Phase of Healing

The inflammatory phase is an essential part of healing, characterised by swelling, pain and heat. It typically lasts several days and plays a crucial role in repairing damaged tissue. However, this phase often goes unnoticed by horse owners, as they cannot see every injury. To effectively treat tissue injuries, prompt intervention is key. Cryotherapy methods such as ice packs or cold running water can control pain, protect tissues, reduce swelling and preserve tissue function. If an injury is suspected, many administer non-steroidal anti-inflammatory drugs (NSAIDs) such as phenylbutazone (bute) for pain relief, but this can potentially delay healing. These block the production of pro-inflammatory mediators, including pain, swelling and oedema, all of which are essential components of the inflammatory phase. Moreover, NSAIDs can have side effects such as stomach lining irritation and gastrointestinal symptoms if used regularly, which is particularly concerning for horses with already compromised gastrointestinal systems. While medication may be necessary for pain relief under veterinary advice, you can also consider natural alternatives, especially for long-term management.

Injury detection can be facilitated through palpation and thorough observation. Proper management of the inflammatory phase is crucial to prevent complications. Failure to address it correctly can lead to prolonged inflammation, which makes tissues rigid, less pliable, and more prone to further injury, contributing to back problems in many horses across various equestrian disciplines.

Musculoskeletal therapists in the equine industry often have a difficult task when they are asked to provide therapy on a horse because it might not be performing as it once did or its movements are not as fluid, often because the injury has been there for some time and was not treated from the outset, thus resulting in further tissue degeneration, which can be more challenging to treat and bring a less positive longer-term outcome for the horse.

Therapeutic Recommendations During the Inflammatory Phase

Cryotherapy to control swelling and pain, but pain relief may be necessary depending on the extent of the injury.

Rest protects the tissues from further damage, so the horse is not moving its body when in pain.

Manual therapy and pain-free movement are intended to preserve function. It would be performed once the inflammation phase is nearing completion using gentle techniques such as effleurage, with some gentle in-hand walking.

The stages of tissue healing are complex and fragile processes. However, if the inflammatory phase is recognised and treated correctly, then it is likely that the other phases of tissue healing can take effect. This would minimise chronic conditions for the horse and a high rate of re-injury occurrence. Therefore, understanding all three critical phases and how to work with your horses during them is very important for long-term outcomes.

Proliferation Phase of Healing

The next phase is known as the proliferation phase, which typically occurs after the completion of the inflammatory phase and can last between four to twenty-four days. During this phase, the muscle tissue or wound undergoes reconstruction with the formation of new tissue, primarily composed of collagen. As new tissues are being formed, the tissue contracts, causing it to shorten and tighten. However, it remains susceptible to re-injury. A new network of blood vessels is also developed to ensure that the granulation tissue, which is vital for healing, receives sufficient oxygen and nutrients. The granulation tissue may be visible outside of the wound, while the damaged muscle lies beneath it, particularly in the case of open wounds.

During this healing phase, the injured tissue is weaker than the adjacent normal tissue, making it vulnerable to re-injury if the horse's movements and manual therapy are not appropriately monitored. The objective is to enhance circulation, encourage collagen alignment, and prevent adhesion formation, which can lead to the formation of rigid and less pliable scar tissue. Scar tissue can impede the horse's movements, causing a restricted range of motion.

Therapeutic Recommendations During the Proliferation Phase

Carefully increase the movement of the horse with in-hand walking.

Gentle manual therapy techniques such as compression, shaking, myofascial release and effleurage.

Remodelling Phase of Healing

The remodelling phase is a critical stage in the healing process for horses following an injury. This phase typically occurs after the inflammatory and proliferation phases and can last for weeks to months, even up to two years, depending on the severity and nature of the injury. During the remodelling phase, the focus shifts from the initial repair of the injured tissue to the restructuring and strengthening of the newly formed tissue. The main goal of this phase is to enhance the functional capacity and integrity of the healed area. As well as the reorganisation of collagen fibres to help to enhance the strength and resilience of the healed tissue, the phase also involves the removal of excessive scar tissue and the maturation of the healed area. Blood vessels and nerve fibres are also restored.

It is important to note that the remodelling phase is a gradual and dynamic process. The newly formed tissue continues to adapt and remodel in response to mechanical stresses. As such, manual therapy can increase the tissue's elasticity, providing more flexibility and range of motion around joints. Often tendons and ligaments re-injure at this phase, due to the horse being exercised too early or incorrectly.

Therapeutic Recommendations During the Remodelling Phase

A gentle and planned return to activity involving gradual rehabilitation exercise to avoid re-injure.

Manual therapy techniques such as friction over adhesion or scar tissue to help elongate the fibres and myofascial release to help stretch the fascia and the muscle can be very beneficial.

HEALTH AND SAFETY CONSIDERATIONS WHEN PERFORMING MANUAL THERAPY

Interacting with horses in any capacity can be risky, and it is crucial to observe basic horse safety guidelines and specific ones when performing manual therapy. This is because you will be working in close proximity to a large animal that may react if you touch a painful area. Here are some specific tips to keep in mind to minimise the risk of injuries.

Environment and Preparation

- Try to perform your therapy when the environment is peaceful, to avoid the horse being startled when in a deep state of relaxation due to the effects of manual therapy by inducing parasympathetic state.
- Avoid other animals in the vicinity – such as dogs, cats and chickens – so there is maximum concentration by both you and the horse.
- Ensure the stable is free from obstacles such as protruding nails and yard tools.
- Avoid a stable with a low beam, where the horse might hit its head if it reacts by throwing it up.
- Remove wet bedding to avoid any potential slipping.
- If you need to stand on a platform to reach the horse, use something sturdy and horse-friendly with no sharp edges; buckets and tack boxes are not safe to use.
- In cold conditions, quarter a warm rug over the horse as you work on different areas.

Specifics for You

- Remove any rings that might scratch the horse, and your fingernails should not be long.
- Wear sturdy stable yard footwear and loose clothing to move freely.
- Avoid wearing a heavy scent because horses can react to certain smells (I know this through my Zoopharmacognosy training).
- Stretch your body beforehand and wear supports if needed.
- Maintain a good posture – keeping the spine straight, shoulders relaxed, and core engaged. Bend

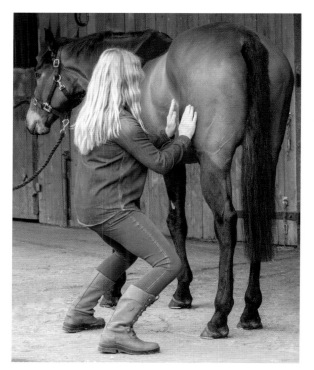

This posture is feet hip-width apart. Keep your back straight with relaxed shoulders and core engaged. Avoid hunching over the horse or twisting your body.

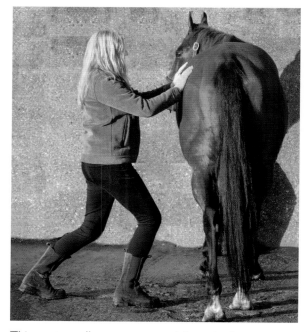

This posture allows you to work into the horse more with an upright upper body posture and one leg in front, which is the working leg, and one behind, which is the support.

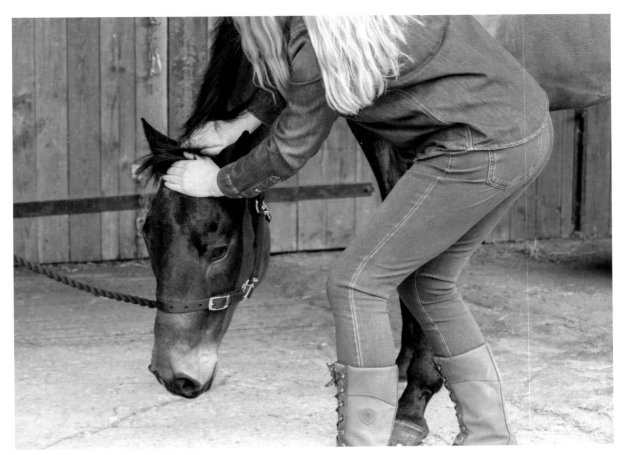

If the horse responds to what you are doing in a way that you might not expect, you need to be able to adjust your posture so you go with the horse and do not spoil the moment. As long as you remain comfortable, your posture can be flexible.

from the knees and use body weight down to the feet instead of relying solely on your upper body strength to minimise the risk of strain or injury during treatments.

- Stand balanced with your feet shoulder-width apart and your weight evenly distributed. This applies to the two stances we use, feet side by side or one behind the other. This assists with your stability.
- Use your body weight instead of your arm strength to apply pressure during the massage.
- Be aware of your breathing and keep it steady and relaxed. If you start to tire, simply take a break to rest your body to avoid fatigue and injury. If possible, remain with your hands resting on the horse so it does not think the session has finished.

- Avoid stretching to perform a technique, use a well-balanced step to stand on with four points of contact with the ground if you need to be in a higher position, such as when working over the back or upper section of the hindquarters.
- If your body parts ache, you are not relaxing them whilst massaging or breathing properly to fuel your muscles. Adjust your positioning and breathing.
- As with all exercise, your body will adapt to massaging your horse the more you practise it.
- Maintaining good physical fitness is also important for overall posture and wellbeing.
- Relax, breathe slowly and deeply and keep your voice low.

Specifics for Your Horse

- The horse should be clean and dry, not dirty, wet or sweating.
- Tie the horse loosely with a lead rope and a well-fitting head collar.
- Ensure the horse has access to hay and fresh, clean water.
- Do not plan the session for at least one-and-a-half hours after the horse has eaten any concentrated feed, or two hours is safest, as this could induce colic. Forage is fine.
- Allocate around one-and-a-half hours maximum for the session, as some horses tend to fidget as the time increases beyond one hour.
- After the session, allow the horse time to relax in the stable or quiet paddock unless you have performed a sports massage (pre-competition).

Contraindications

A contraindication is a reason you would not perform manual therapy on a horse because it may be harmful or interact negatively with a specific situation, drug, procedure or surgery. The following is a list of contra-indications you must be aware of:

- If the horse is unwell and not its usual self.
- If severe diarrhoea or an unknown cause of any nasal discharge is present.
- Fever, viral disease or infection present, including influenza, herpes and strangles.
- Skin conditions such as ringworm, sore areas and open wounds.
- If an abscess is present.
- Severe acute physical injury or trauma such as in-flammation, bleeding, a broken bone, a fracture or tendon injury. With mild to moderate muscle injuries, follow the muscle injury-specific strategies.
- Malignant tumours or any condition that could spread.
- During treatment with antibiotics.
- Following a vaccination.
- After hard work until all vital signs have normalised.
- A wet or sweating horse.

- If the horse is in shock or suffering from fatigue or exhaustion.
- A very lame horse that has not seen a veterinarian.

Also, you should not massage a mare in the first three months of pregnancy. Although during the pregnancy, it should be acceptable and very benefi-cial, providing the veterinarian has no concerns with the mare, and you do not perform any stimulating techniques as this could divert blood away from the foal and also a possibility to carry metabolic waste from the mare to the placenta. However, gentle com-pression or shaking techniques or myofascial release should be fine in normal pregnancy circumstances.

Contra-actions

Contra-actions are reactions to manual therapy that are not necessarily negative; they might occur or never happen. As you will be monitoring the horse during and after the session, you should be able to identify if the horse has experienced a contra-action so you can consider this for your next session. Exam-ples of contra-actions:

- Fatigue that occurs after the release of a toxin build-up.
- Heightened emotional state due to the positive re-lease from deep-held feelings and emotions.
- Frequent need to drink fresh, clean water and to urinate due to stimulation of the lymphatic system.
- Active bowel movements, as all body systems tend to work more optimally.

If a negative contra-action occurs during the treat-ment, you must stop: such as the horse starting to sweat that is not in response to ambient temperature; the horse shivering when the environment is not cold; appearing unsteady or lightheaded or wanting to lie down. In addition, if the horse becomes very agitated and restless with negative behaviour towards you, this indicates the horse is unhappy with what you are doing; you either need to adjust the techniques you are using and, if that does not work, stop altogether and reassess the horse. I must note, in all my years of working with horses in this way, I have never seen a negative contra-action – but that is not to say you will not.

HOW BEST TO PROGRESS WITH THE MANUAL THERAPY

Once you are ready to start, you need to be open-minded to respond to the horse's needs during the therapy rather than following a systematic routine, because you may need to adjust what you are doing or find a more appropriate technique.

The initial contact with the horse is vital for a successful therapy session. You should always enter the stable calmly, in a non-forceful manner. The horse needs to feel safe and trust you from the beginning and learn that you will not groom or tack the horse to ride it; this is something different you do with it. This not only applies when you are performing therapy with the horse; out of respect for the horse and the fact that you are entering the horse's space, you should always adopt this approach.

As the horse relaxes, its muscles will also relax, which benefits the therapy and the outcome. You will not get good results working on a tense horse.

Observe the horse in the stable, giving you current information about how the horse is feeling.

What are its demeanour and behaviour indicating?

Does it appear to be eating and drinking usually?

Does its toileting look normal?

Is it standing squarely and moving around the stable fluidly?

Is its posture normal, head, neck, back, hindquarters and limbs?

Are there any signs of injury to its body or the stable?

Are there any swellings to its body or excess body fluids such as watery eyes, nasal discharge, diarrhoea or blood?

Are there any contraindications present – reasons you would not provide manual therapy?

If you intend to proceed, then loosely tie the horse, so it can express itself or manoeuvre during the session or you can work with your horse untied if you know the horse well or it is accustomed to having manual therapy.

Keep a hay net in easy reach so the horse can nibble – which they often like – and have access to clean water. If the horse is loosely tied but unable to reach its water bucket, you need to have a break after fifteen minutes so the horse can drink if required. But no feed or treats are allowed.

Talk to the horse in a calm and quiet voice, which will help you to understand how the horse is feeling and reacting to your touch. There is a definite exchange of energy when working with a horse; the more positive the energy from you, the better.

Work in a slow, methodical manner and not too deeply. Many horses prefer a lighter touch, but you will gauge what your horse likes, as they all differ. Monitor the horse's body reactions to what you are doing, always being mindful of negative and positive reactions so you can adjust accordingly.

If your horse is enjoying what you are doing, and most horses do, watch for the positive signs such as heavy eyes, blinking, staring, closing eyes, deeper breathing, sighing, lowering the head, lowering or quivering bottom lip, licking and chewing, shaking the head, rolling back the eye, stretching and even

★ TOP TIP

This is valuable time spent with the horse, and you will find that the more manual therapy you provide, the more the horse will look forward to it as a time when it can relax with you and not be expected to perform for you. The more therapy sessions you undertake on your horse, you will find that your relationship is enhanced, as it is also a time when you can reward it for all your horse does for you. This is a therapeutic time for the horse, and your undivided attention will help them relax and benefit fully from the therapy.

yawning. Ensure the horse can yawn if it needs to, by wearing a loose headcollar that allows the jaw to open fully. Often the horse will move its body into you as you work on an area it particularly likes, or it will keep looking at an area as if to ask you to go there. You might also find that the horse stands very still with a stare, another sign that it is processing the therapy.

Be aware of the ambient temperature; if the horse is getting warm, allow more breaks; if it starts to sweat, stop what you are doing. If it is a cold day, quarter the sections you are not working on with a rug. It is best to avoid manual therapy in extremes of temperature, either very hot or cold.

It is crucial to keep your attention focused solely on the horse during the session and not allow other people or animals to be a distraction. In addition, try to avoid planning these sessions around busy yard times when other people might be coming and going, such as farrier visits, feed times, bringing horses in or turning them out, as this will affect the quality of the therapy.

You should already know whether your horse is auditory – one that pays more attention to sounds; if so, it will listen and react to sounds, so it is essential to talk to this type of horse to encourage relaxation and preferably house it in a stable that is not in a busy or noisy area, because they like peace. Your horse might be a visual one that reacts more to sights and is better housed and treated in a stable away from lots of visual activity.

Afterwards

Besides a pre-competition massage, you should keep the horse quiet and comfortable and allow it to process the manual therapy after slowly walking in hand for a few minutes, providing the environment is quiet and any distractions will not undo the relaxation you have created. This is not essential, but I do find some horses benefit from a gentle walk. Then, leave the horse peacefully in the stable for a while and then turn out, or it can stay in its stable if the massage is performed late in the day and is usually stabled overnight.

If your therapy has been a post-competition massage, maintenance or remedial, then it is beneficial to allow the horse to rest afterwards for at least 48 hours. However, in some circumstances, 24 hours will be sufficient. The longer the rest period, the more beneficial it is for the horse, but this depends on its fitness, what level of schooling and competition it is at, and so on.

The horse may be thirstier than usual, so ensure plenty of fresh, clean water is available. This helps to expel toxins. They also like to nibble on forage after a massage.

The following day, the horse may be sore if the massage caused an inflammatory response, if there are any underlying injuries, or if the horse might still be processing the therapy and feeling the benefit. It is, therefore, advisable to give the horse turnout but no ridden exercise unless you have performed a pre-competition massage.

After the manual therapy, you will have the opportunity to assess the horse's reactions, whether it highlighted any concerns for you in terms of specific aftercare and management it might need, for example:

- Does the bit, bridle, girth or saddle need to be checked?
- Do you need to reassess the use of training aids?
- Do you need some musculoskeletal therapy or ridden coaching?
- Do you need to alter the training programme and schedule?
- Does the horse need to be ridden in less flexion?
- Did the horse appear to have any digestive discomfort? You might need to refer to an independent nutritionist or a veterinarian to rule out gastric or colonic conditions.
- Does the horse need dental attention or farriery?
- Is the environment suitable for the horse? do you think the horse is happy where he is currently housed, or could some changes be made which are more beneficial to its wellbeing?

Stretching Horses

Note: Although stretching horses seems popular among many professionals, I disagree with it – especially for horse owners to perform. As such, there are no stretches in this book.

Gentle passive stretching can be applied during a rehabilitation situation by a professional therapist, as guided by the injury and the veterinarian, if involved. However, horse owners should not perform stretching daily nor when girthing the horse, when little is known about the underlying structures. We see images throughout the media of horses being stretched into unnatural positions that they would not do themselves. These are over-complicated and, if done in the wrong circumstances or incorrectly, can be very harmful to the horse.

When you stretch yourself, you know exactly when to stop, which is when it hurts, but a horse being stretched does not have that choice. As such, more problems can result in the horse being stretched. Baited stretches, such as using a carrot to entice a horse into a position, are considered outdated and damaging. The horse will do anything for a treat, which may mean it is overstretching a body part to reach the treat and causing damage.

The main reasons not to stretch your horse are:

- Horse owners do not have the extensive required anatomy training.
- The tissue might not be pliable enough, which also carries the risk of tearing any injured tissue and healthy tissue.
- The stretch can be performed incorrectly.
- There may be an underlying undiagnosed condition that would render a stretch a contraindication.
- There may be a loose piece of bone or fracture that can be dislodged during a stretch or damaged further.
- A horse should not need stretching before work; sufficient warm-up and cool-down during the sessions should sufficiently prepare the tissues.

Leave stretching to the horse; the horse can control how far it needs to stretch to reach that itch or that plant that looks inviting over the fence. It is doubtful that the horse will intentionally hurt itself trying to stretch, as it knows when to stop.

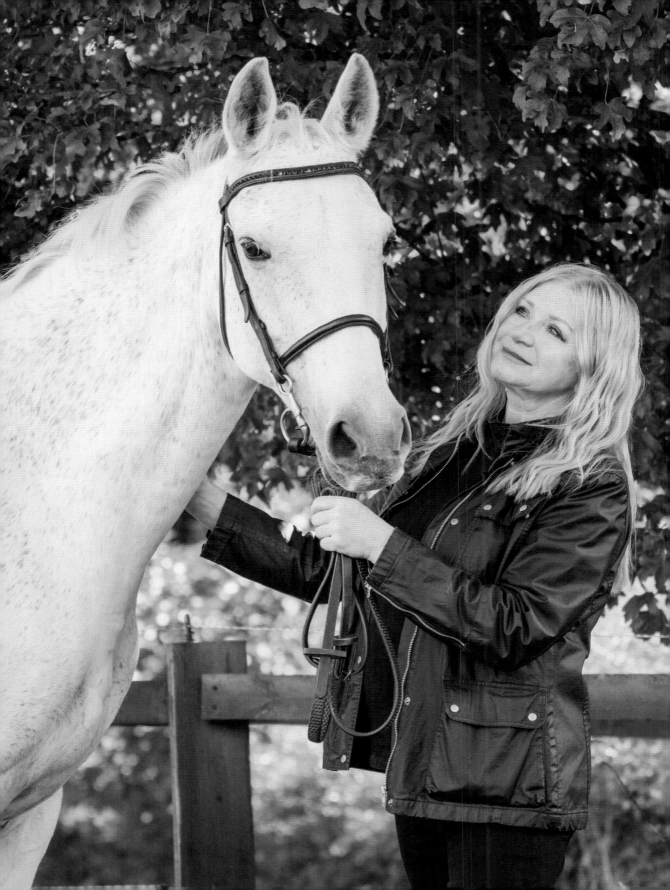

PART II – PRACTICE

CHAPTER 6

Palpation, Detecting Pain or Abnormality

The Palpation Examination

Before embarking on any manual therapy with your horse, you need to thoroughly palpate first, which is a method of feeling over the contours of its body with your hands to perform a physical examination. Your palpation examination is to detect any pain or abnormality in the muscle tissues, changes from a pliable muscle to that which has tension and might contain adhesions or knots, spasms, tears, restrictions in the fascia and so on. It is also used to gauge your horse's level of sensitivity and whether pain might be present.

The main difference between a professional musculoskeletal therapist palpating a horse and a horse owner is the level of training and expertise. The professional should have received specialised training in the anatomy and physiology of horses and how to assess and address issues related to their musculoskeletal system. They have a deep understanding of the biomechanics of horse movement and are trained to identify areas of tension, restriction or dysfunction through palpation and other diagnostic techniques.

In contrast, a horse owner may not have the same level of training or experience in assessing their horse's musculoskeletal health. While they may be familiar with their horse's general movement and behaviour, they may not have the same level of knowledge when it comes to identifying specific areas of tension or dysfunction and may not be able to detect more subtle problems.

As such, I am going to provide you with step-by-step instructions on how to palpate your horse's muscles so that you will become more proficient at it, the more you do it.

During palpation, you are monitoring what you are feeling and the horse's reactions to your touch. By the time you have completed your entire palpation on both sides of the horse's body, you will have a focus on where you want to apply your manual therapy to support your horse. It might be mid-neck, across the back, to the hamstring muscles – it might be all over. It might be the same on the other side, but it might be different.

Continuously monitor your horse's reactions during the palpation examination: the rule of thumb is that if the horse is happy with the palpation, it will show positive signs such as sighing, closing or blinking his eyes, working into you as you palpate, lowering its head, just as the horse would when enjoying receiving manual therapy. If the horse is not comfortable, it will give negative signs such as flinching, moving away from you, tail swishing and so on; then, stop what you are doing or ease off with the pressure. You might be palpating too firmly for the horse, or you have found a very tender area.

In order to assess a horse's musculoskeletal health

effectively, it is important to pay attention not only to their reactions but also to the muscles and tissues under your hand. Experienced equine and human therapists use 'temperature, texture, tenderness, and tension' to evaluate the horse's condition. By feeling for these four indicators, therapists can get a better understanding of any areas of tension, pain or dysfunction and tailor their treatment accordingly.

TEMPERATURE

An average body temperature of a horse is 38 degrees celsius. If an area is abnormally cold, it suggests a lack of blood supply, so there could be a nerve entrapment. If it is unusually hot, it indicates inflammation and possibly a condition in the under-lying tissues or an injury.

Temperature changes can be caused by a variety of reasons, including:

- Exercise can cause muscles to generate heat due to the increased metabolic activity required to meet the demands of the activity. This can cause a tem-porary increase in muscle temperature. As such, ensure you do not palpate your horse immediately after exercise.
- Inflammatory conditions, such as muscle strains or tears, can cause an increase in muscle tempera-ture due to the release of inflammatory chemicals.
- Nerve damage can affect a horse's ability to reg-ulate muscle temperature, leading to fluctuations in temperature. Usually, a nerve impingement in an area will feel unusually cold.
- Bone conditions such as arthritis can cause changes in temperature.
- Infections, such as certain bacterial or viral, can cause an increase in muscle temperature due to the release of pyrogens, which are substances that cause fever. You would not be palpating your horse with a view to providing manual therapy if an infection was present for risk of spreading. This would be a contraindication referred to in Chapter 5.

TEXTURE

Healthy muscle tissue should feel pliable with elasticity. With regular, correct exercise and rest, a horse's muscles should become more firm and toned. Conversely, muscle tissue that is too soft, has atrophy, feels weak or has swelling (oedema), means the horse is not working evenly and has imbalances or an injury which will need manual therapy and correct supportive exercise. It could also indicate a sluggish circulatory system, which manual therapy would assist.

You might feel some firm bands of tissue within the muscle. These are adhesions whereby the muscle fibres are stuck together, causing a restriction in the horse's movement. Even if the adhesion is small, it will stop that muscle from contracting and relaxing as it should and can hurt the horse.

A variety of reasons cause texture changes, including:

- Aging horses can lose tone to their muscles and become softer and atrophy, which results in a texture change.
- Injuries to the muscles can cause swelling and tenderness.
- Certain diseases such as equine polysaccharide storage myopathy (EPSM) or hyperkalemic pe-riodic paralysis (HYPP), can cause changes in muscle texture, such as stiffness or weakness.
- Hormonal imbalances, such as those associated with Cushing's disease, can cause changes in muscle texture.
- Dehydration, which can cause the coat to feel dry and the muscles to move slowly under your hand.
- Hypertonicity indicated by taut muscle fibres with little or no pliability.

You will become more adept at knowing what is normal and what is not as you regularly palpate and provide manual therapy on your horse. However, if you suspect any texture changes in your horse's muscles that might be disease-related, contact a musculoskeletal therapist or your veterinarian.

TENDERNESS

This is the degree to which your horse responds to your touch. You cannot necessarily feel tenderness; it is your horse's reaction to your touch, it will let you know if where you are palpating is tender.

If highly sensitive, it may indicate tension and pain in the muscle, or nerve endings may be irritated. The horse's reaction to your touch suggests how severe the underlying condition is. This is likely caused by overtraining, incorrect exercise, incorrect use of training aids, rider asymmetry, and tack not being comfortable for the horse. The horse could also be tender around the abdomen if it has gastrointestinal discomfort.

TENSION

Too much tension, also known as hypertonicity or when the muscles become overly contracted, can be due to a variety of reasons, including:

- Overexertion or overuse when the horse is asked to perform strenuous activities without proper conditioning and rest it can develop tense muscles.
- Overuse of training aids that block the horse's natural movement, causing the muscles to work incorrectly and develop tension.
- Injury or pain from a strain, sprain, adhesion or tear may develop tension around the area and possibly in adjacent muscles as they are asked to work harder when the tense muscle tries to protect itself. This can also cause compensation movement patterns.
- Incorrect saddle fit can cause discomfort and tension in the horse's back and shoulder muscles.
- An unlevel rider can cause tension in the horse's muscles as it tries to compensate in its movements for the asymmetry generated from the rider.
- Incorrect bit/bridle or fit or dental problems can cause discomfort and tension in the horse's neck and jaw muscles.
- Nutritional imbalances – the horse requires a balanced diet for its muscles to function correctly. If a

horse is deficient in specific nutrients or consumes an imbalanced diet, it can lead to tense muscles.
- Stress or anxiety can cause a horse to develop tense muscles due to holding their bodies in a tense posture.

★ TOP TIP

There is a lot to think about as you embark on learning the skill of palpating your horse. However, in time you will learn to listen to the muscles as they will tell you a story and, as you palpate: make a mental note of what the muscle or the horse is communicating to you; start to think about what you do with the horse in terms of its training, your riding technique, the last time you had its tack checked and so on. You are potentially looking for the cause of that temperature, texture, tenderness or muscle tension change. Keep practising – your skills will develop over time and if you do suspect the horse is displaying something more than your manual therapy skills can help, then seek support from a professional therapist.

How to Perform the Palpation

You will follow the direction of the horse's coat when palpating by adopting a smooth stroking-type movement over the entire body with a flat to slightly cupped hand. There is no need to prod or poke; you shape your hand to the body's contours and apply a light to moderate pressure, slightly more than stroking your horse. When palpating, you have a definite goal: to examine the tissues, giving you your therapy focus. Your palpation is very unlike veterinary palpation. When a veterinarian deeply palpates a horse with an instrument, it is usually to ascertain a neurological response, not the integrity of the muscles, which is your focus.

Some sources will tell you to apply a particular pressure, but I find this unhelpful, as every horse is different, so the pressure you use will differ; some are more ticklish than others, some like a firmer pressure, whilst some like it gentle. Also, a finer-skinned thoroughbred might require less pressure than a thicker-skinned cob. With these variances in mind, you need to gauge what is acceptable for your horse, only applying sufficient pressure during palpation for you to receive a subtle reaction. Of course, if the horse is uncomfortable and you apply too much pressure to an area where it is tender, then it will react negatively. This does not accurately represent proper palpation, because you have elicited a response by working too deeply. If you stroke the horse all over first and monitor its reaction, then often palpation is not much deeper than stroking it.

THE HEAD

The horse's head is large and elongated, with a long muzzle and large nostrils that help it to breathe more easily during physical activity. The horse's eyes are on the sides of its head, giving it a wide field of vision and the ability to detect predators and other potential threats. The ears are also large and mobile, allowing the horse to hear and focus on sounds from all directions. We should not restrict any of these body parts, as they are part of the horse's sensory apparatus, which it relies on for survival. Tight bridles, some training aids or bits, hoods and blinkers would all constitute a restriction.

The Forehead

The forehead is the area between and just above the eyes. Foreheads can be concave, flat or convex. The hollow above the eyes is the sub-orbital depression. In most well-cared-for horses, this will be a shallow depression. Older horses, or those with less well care, will have a very deep sub-orbital depression.

Starting with the horse's forehead can be helpful to assess whether the horse has a tension headache caused by its environment, training, tack or rider. It is important to palpate gently and carefully to avoid causing discomfort or pain for the horse, as the

forehead is a sensitive area. You will also see if the muscles are developing evenly; if not, the horse might not be chewing correctly. It is also a good indicator of bridle fit.

You might also look at the horse's eyes and check if they are they in balance; if not, there could be tension in the muscle above one eye that looks higher and tighter than the other eye. If there is tension, think about what you are doing as a rider with your hands on the side with tension, is that your dominant side? Also, the horse might need dental attention, particularly to the tense side, as the forehead muscles are a good indicator of chewing and dental health. Above the eyes are the sub-orbital depression and, if filled, can indicate the presence of a metabolic condition which might need veterinarian advice.

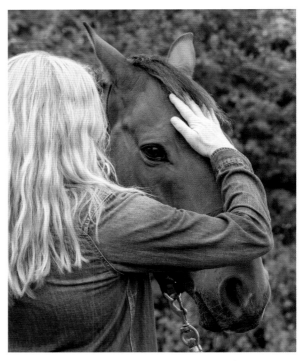

Start by placing your hand in the centre of the horse's forehead. It might resist this initially as you will be in an area of 'personal space'. Stay here for a few moments so the horse gets used to you being there. Then slowly palpate up the centre of the forehead using your entire hand and fingers, finishing at the base of the forelock. Repeat to the left and right sides toward the base of each ear.

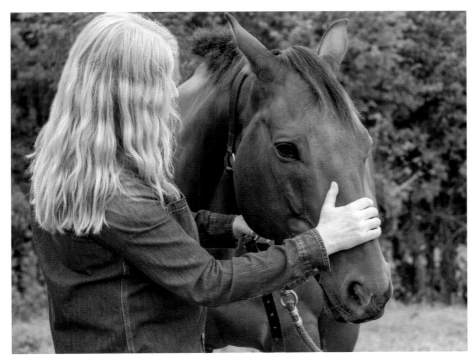

Cup the nasal bone in the palm of your hand and starting just below the eyes, palpate all the way to the end of the nose. Despite its size, this is a very fragile bone that can injure very easily.

The Nasal Bone

Palpating the horse's nasal bone is next and will indicate if the horse has any tension from the noseband, sinus pain, other nerve pain or a potential issue with the respiratory system. If there is tenderness present, there could be inflammation in the area, and the horse might have trouble breathing through a nostril or have an infection. Tenderness to the area of the noseband implies it is too tight or not placed correctly; often, nosebands are too low, impinging on nerves.

If you are in a secure enclosure, you can remove the head collar to allow you better access and not risk getting your hand trapped under the headcollar, especially if the horse is tender and flinches or raises its head quickly. This applies to all face palpations.

The Jaw

The horse's jaw is large and powerful, with strong cheek muscles used for chewing and grinding food (masseter m.). When palpating the cheek, if you feel tension here or the horse flinches and exhibits tenderness, then you would need to check the bit; the

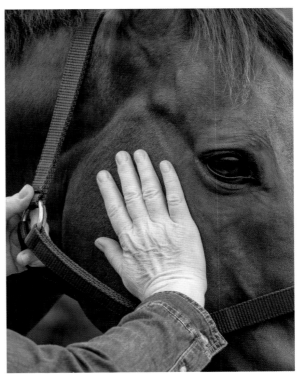

Palpate the entire cheek area with a flat hand; palpate upwards, then circle around the mandible (jaw) edge and repeat.

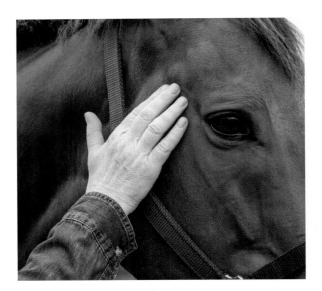

Palpate the TMJ by positioning your fingertips directly on the hinge of the joint and remain there for a few moments, continue by gently palpating the entire joint.

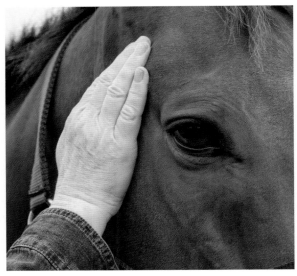

Place your hand gently over the TMJ area and maintain contact. Watch the horse's eye soften and possibly close, indicating relief. This signals the horse's discomfort, which you acknowledge by staying on the area.

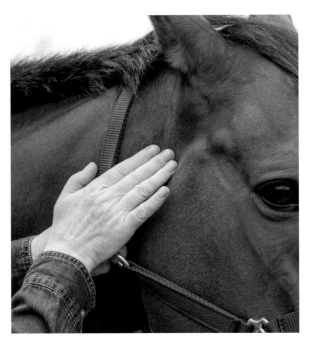

Starting just above my fingers, level with the eye, gently palpate downwards in the space to the edge of the jaw and monitor the horse's reaction. You should be able to place two fingers in the space. Repeat on the other side. Check if they are the same. If not, the horse's tack, riding style and teeth need assessing.

muscles can become tense due to gripping onto or avoiding a bit; the bridle fit, and consider what you do with your hands when riding and your balance; also, dental attention might be required.

The Temporomandibular Joint (TMJ)

The TMJ is the joint that connects the horse's skull to its jawbone and allows the horse to open and close its mouth. Palpating the TMJ can help identify any joint discomfort, inflammation or misalignments. It can also reveal information about the horse's dental health and comfort whilst eating and when being ridden.

The Interspace

The interspace between the neck and the head is very important, contributing to flexion, extension, lateral flexion and some slight axial rotation movement. You should be able to place two fingers in the space on both sides of the horse. This area can suffer from tension and inflammation from horses being ridden in too much head flexion and from poorly fitting tack and training aids or rider hands locking the horse's head into position.

THE NECK

The Poll and Upper Cervical

Next, palpate around the poll and upper cervical area (the atlas and the axis joints). These landmarks are located in the upper part of the neck where the horse's skull meets its neck – important for supporting the horse's head and the muscles around the poll for flexion and extension of the neck.

Common causes of tension here are poor riding or training aids, poorly fitting tack such as a tight browband or headband and underlying musculoskeletal issues. For example, if the rider is pulling too hard on the reins, using a bit that is incorrect or too severe, or locking the horse's head in with training aids, the horse will develop tension or pain in these joints and muscles. Other possible causes of poll, atlas and axis joint tension include injuries or neck trauma, dental issues, and underlying medical conditions such as arthritis or degenerative joint disease. High hay net positioning can also contribute to tension in this region.

If your palpation reveals tension, then you must follow a process of elimination to find the root cause; then, treatment may involve initial rest, manual therapy and correct supportive exercise.

The Cervical Neck

The neck is long and flexible, consisting of seven cervical vertebrae that allow for a wide range of movement. The neck muscles are powerful and provide the horse with excellent balance and control over its head and body – another reason the horse should be allowed to use its neck naturally and not be held in place by hands or training aids. Holding it in places extra strain on the rest of the body, as it searches for balance and stability from elsewhere in the body when the neck is not allowed to perform its role.

A horse's neck can develop muscle problems for various reasons, including physical strain, poor posture, improper training and underlying health issues. Physical strain results from overuse and repetitive movements such as bending, turning or pulling. This can lead to tightness or stiffness in the muscles and connective

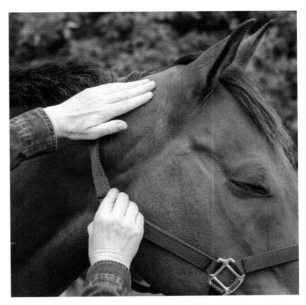

Place your hand behind the poll and maintain gentle pressure until the horse relaxes. If the horse shows resistance, it suggests pain, so continue while speaking softly to the horse. This horse closes its eye, indicating tenderness in that area which needs addressing. As you palpate, gradually glide your hand along the neck, moving over the atlas and axis at the upper area to approximately the midpoint of the neck.

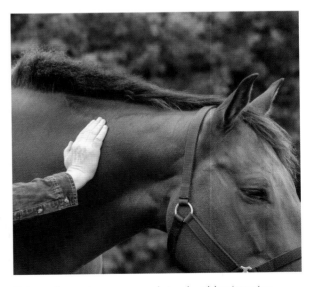

Palpate from the upper neck to shoulder junction, including: crest, middle and lower sections. Also, palpate the underside. Observe the horse's reactions, such as moving towards or away, indicating tension. In the image, the horse experiences relief as its eyes close.

tissues of the neck. The equestrian discipline is usually a contributing factor, along with improper training, incorrect or strong bits, overuse of training aids such as side reins, incorrect riding position and rider's hands.

If the horse spends too much time with its head raised when in a stable and not enough down whilst grazing, it can cause neck tension in the muscles and tendons, leading to discomfort. Again, management practices are likely to be the cause.

The Crest

The crest of the neck should feel strong but pliable with no noticeable contours – that is, thicker parts or atrophied areas that indicate a problem in the muscle. The crest can have tension for a variety of factors: poor riding technique or balance causes the horse to brace against the rider's hands, and tension develops in the neck and crest. Improper training and the use of training aids can affect the crest. Also, back pain and tension can generate forward into the neck and crest, and head pain too. Considering behaviour, horses suffering from anxiety or stress tend to hold tension in their crest also.

The practice of artificially creating 'cresty' necks in horses through various methods such as overfeeding, under-exercising, and hormone supplementation is often done for aesthetic purposes in the showing industry. However, this practice can lead to serious health issues for the horse, including insulin resistance, laminitis and other metabolic disorders such as equine metabolic syndrome (EMS) and Cushing's disease. Additionally, artificially creating 'cresty' necks prioritises aesthetics over the health and welfare of the horses, which goes against my principles of responsible equine husbandry. Therefore, I do not condone this practice in the showing industry.

You will not be able to correctly palpate a horse's crest if it has evidence of excessive fat deposits.

THE SHOULDER

The horse's shoulder plays a critical role in its movement, as it connects its front leg to its body and is responsible for supporting the weight of the horse's front end. During movement, the horse's shoulder allows for the extension and flexion of the front leg, which helps the horse to step forward and push off the ground. The shoulder also provides shock absorption as the horse's front legs make contact with the ground.

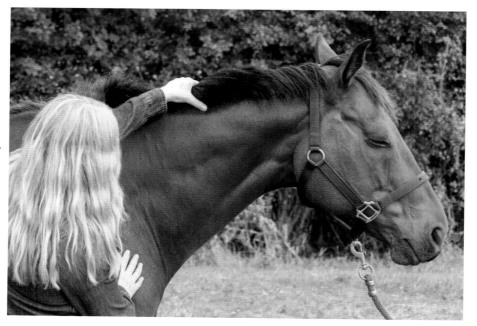

Slowly palpate in a 'scooping' motion whereby the crest of the neck is between your fingers and thumb and held in your hand; starting at the withers finishing as far as you can go on the crest near the poll area, moving in a steady pace. You might feel some texture changes.

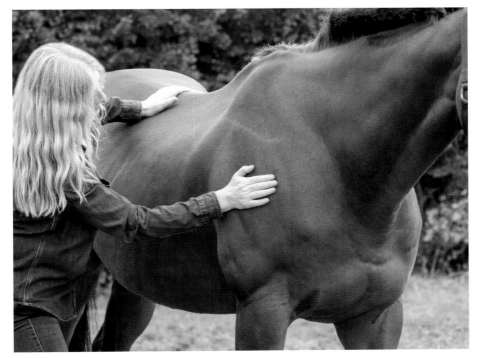

Begin at the withers and palpate the front edge towards the shoulder's meeting point with the front limb. Proceed down the shoulder's midline, passing through the triceps muscles and reaching the top of the leg. Finally, palpate along the back edge, from the withers towards the horse's elbow near the girth area. The shoulder area encompasses a larger space than is commonly perceived.

Any reaction to shoulder palpation will give you information about the horse's movement patterns and the concussion it receives from various riding surfaces – especially the extremes, too firm or too soft, and whether the horse does a lot of jumping, as this causes tension in the shoulder muscles and the bones too from the impact of concussion through the front feet, limbs and then into the shoulder. As a result of the concussion, the triceps muscle at the lower end of the shoulder above the forelimb can be very tender.

Injuries in the shoulder such as from a fall or sudden wrong movements, can develop as tension in the shoulder. For example, muscle strain from overuse or lack of correct training and poor riding technique, or a rider who pulls too hard on the reins or puts too much weight onto the horse's front end, causes shoulder tension. Incorrect saddle fit or sitting it too far forward can place pressure on the horse's shoulders and block shoulder movement resulting in tension. The saddle should sit two-finger width behind the shoulder.

The shoulder will also absorb more tension if the horse is ridden or lunged on the forehand.

THE BACK

The horse's back is a crucial anatomical feature that allows for the placement of a saddle and rider. It also plays an important role in the horse's movement and balance, as it is the foundation of the horse's spine and core. It can react to palpation mainly due to incorrect saddle and girth fit. This can be very damaging over time, causing pressure points in the muscles and adhesions, which are often found on palpation. In addition, an asymmetrical rider, poor riding technique, sitting too heavy in the saddle or poor mounting can cause the back to spasm, which locks the muscle fibres together. Backs can easily bruise because of the additional weight they carry with the rider and tack.

Incorrect training and tack can cause the back muscles to atrophy. You can usually find atrophy as you palpate from behind the shoulder/withers along the back; your hand will drop into a more hollow area (even subtle) rather than glide over an even muscle covering.

Over-training as well as injury, falls, or the horse getting cast in a stable, all result in muscle damage. Also, if the horse lies down in a stable at night and

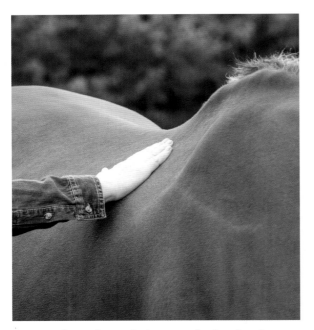

Begin at the withers, placing your flat hand and fingers below the spine, and glide towards the junction where the back meets the hindquarters. Repeat the movement, starting just below where you began, ensuring your wrist goes no further than where the ribs start. Additionally, run your hands over the horse's spine to detect any variations in temperature that could indicate bone damage or degeneration.

there is insufficient bedding – especially those horses bedded on shavings – the horse's body and its back are not correctly supported. Also, the back can become tense from standing in the stable for long periods; horses were meant to keep moving for most of the day, not standing still.

If the horse has an acute muscle condition in its back, it will be tense and tender; if it has a chronic or long-term condition, it will feel rigid, as the horse is 'muscle guarding'; this is a natural physiological response to protect a muscle or an injured area of the body from further harm. It is the involuntary tightening or contraction of the muscles that occurs when there is a perceived threat to the area. The purpose of muscle guarding is to restrict movement and prevent further damage to the affected area. It is unhealthy for a horse to be ridden when it is muscle guarding.

THE RIBS

The ribs are important in the horse's respiratory system and overall physical health. Therefore, any issues with the ribs, such as muscle tension or injury, can affect the horse's breathing, movement, and overall comfort.

The ribs can react to palpation for various reasons, including an incorrectly fitting saddle as it causes pressure on the ribs, and a rider sitting asymmetrically with more weight through their femur. A horse could easily strain one of the intercostal muscles between the ribs due to over-exertion, incorrect movement or sudden trauma. Respiratory issues, such as asthma or heaves, can cause the muscles in the rib area to tense up as the horse works harder to breathe. Also, neurological problems such as spinal cord injury can cause muscle tension and weakness in various parts of the horse's body, including the ribs.

Any reaction to palpation around the ribs might indicate gastrointestinal discomfort also.

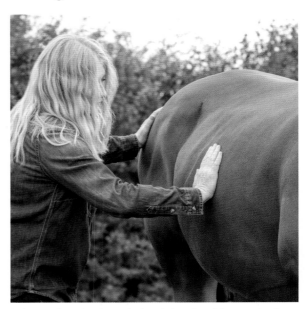

Palpate the ribs from behind the shoulder to the last rib (thoracic eighteen). Repeat again slightly below where you have just palpated – my hand is halfway along this part of the palpation. You will repeat this around four or five times to palpate the ribs entirely, ending at the undercarriage. They are a common site for injury and are often missed.

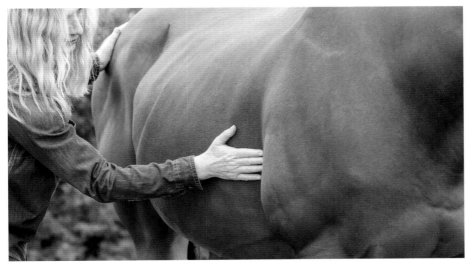

Palpate the entire girth area from behind the shoulder, just below the withers, down to the undercarriage; you may need to repeat a few times, starting very gently and then gradually increasing your palpation pressure because the horse can be quite reactive here. In the image, I am three-quarters of the way down the palpation.

The Girth

The muscles in the girth area, including the pectoral muscles, intercostal muscles and abdominals, are responsible for supporting the horse's body and also play a large part in providing the horse with the necessary strength and flexibility to move freely whilst carrying a rider. However, some horses may develop anxiety around the girth area and react to girth fastening and palpation not only due to pain but past negative experiences causing pain when people tighten girths too quickly and too tightly, thus causing resistance when saddling.

A lot of muscle damage occurs in the girth area, mainly due to incorrect type and fit of the girth and its role in stabilising the saddle, especially if the saddle is not a good fit. I always recommend anatomically-shaped girths over elastic girths that cause muscle damage when fastened too tightly as the horse braces against the pressure from the girth and results in muscle tension. It is also vital to remember that the girth also sits over the breathing apparatus.

You could feel a tissue texture in the girth area that you might not feel elsewhere, such as tears and adhesions that feel like 'elastic bands' or 'bubble wrap' popping under the skin. This indicates there is tension and damage, usually tears and fascial restrictions. This should not be present but, unfortunately, is very common with many horses.

I disagree with the practice of stretching the horse's limb forward when girthing – this is outdated given the construction of girths used today; it was started as a practice to stop elastic girths from nipping the skin. This, however, causes tears in the muscles of the girth area. Gently fastening the girth from the ground should suffice. When a rider is mounted and attempts to tighten the girth further, this causes overtightening because much strength is available when sitting on the horse and pulling up the girth, and as such, overtightening can occur.

The Hindquarters

The hindquarter muscling generates a great deal of force when pushing off from them to move the horse's body forward, and they provide balance and stability when standing and in motion, heavily relied upon for jumping activities and working in collection.

The muscle health in this region will indicate whether the horse is moving correctly, whether there is sacroiliac pain, hamstring pain and so on. The muscles of the hindquarters can have tension and become overdeveloped if the horse is not training correctly or tied in at the hind end with training aids. Conversely, they can be weak or atrophied – especially along the back in the lumbosacral area just in front of the croup, behind where the saddle sits, also in the gluteals and hip flexors when the horse is not correctly engaging its hindquarters.

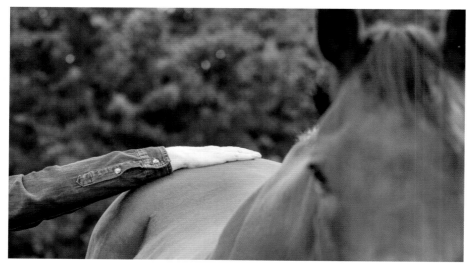

Begin palpation from the croup, where my hand is positioned, just after the lumbar area of the back where you previously finished palpating. Continue the palpation towards the dock and cover all areas in the upper region of the hindquarters. Ensure you thoroughly examine each spot before moving on to the lower section.

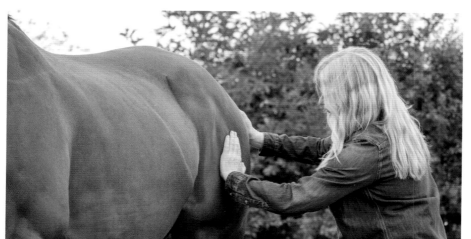

Palpate the hip flexor muscles, ensuring complete coverage of the entire area. Begin just below the tuber coxa (hip bone) and work your way from left to right, following the placement of my hands and finish level with the stifle.

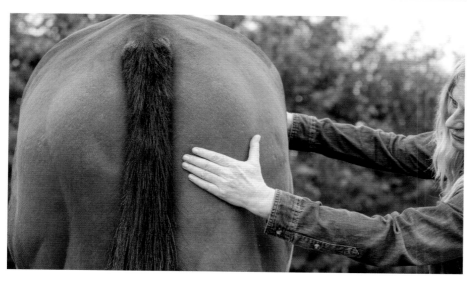

Finally, palpate the hamstring group of muscles, starting alongside the tail and working down towards the hock. Ensure the entire area is covered, the section closest to the tail, the middle section as shown in the image and the outside section.

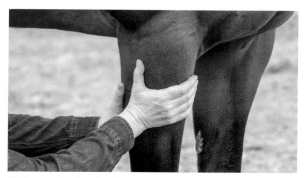

Palpate the forelimbs with your hands on the inside and outside edge of the leg. Palpate from the top of the leg to the carpus (knee) and then again with your hands to the front of the leg and the back, as shown in the image.

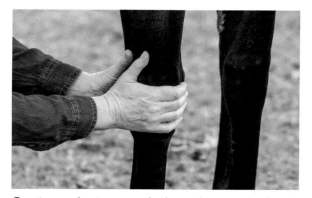

Continue palpating over the knee down to the foot, ensuring you cover the circumference of the knee and all around the metacarpal bone (fore cannon).

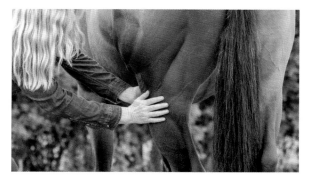

Palpate the muscles of the hindlimb, using one hand inside the limb and the other on the outside, as you move towards the tarsus (hock). Next, examine the front and back of the limb. Proceed from the hock, palpating down the metatarsal bones (hind cannon) all the way to the foot, similar to how you examined the forelimbs.

THE LIMBS

The horse's limb muscles play a key role in its movement and locomotion and these muscles are often overlooked, the focus being mainly on bone, tendon and ligament.

They are small muscles in comparison to others but powerful for generating propulsion as they contract and relax to move the horse's limbs, as well as support the horse's body when standing or in movement, which is a feat, as the horse's body is very heavy. In addition, during galloping or jumping movements, the limb muscles require a great deal of strength, as they do when the horse makes sudden turns or when navigating uneven terrain.

When palpating the limbs, you explore the muscles and bones to identify what is typical for your horse and what is not. For instance, if the horse has a knee-related orthopaedic issue, it may feel cool to the touch due to poor circulation or from standing in the stable for an extended period. Alternatively, the tendons might feel warmer after physical activity.

After completing the limb palpation, you should inspect the feet for symmetry, high heel/low heel, length of the toe, and weight distribution, which dictates how the horse loads its limbs and influences foot growth. Shoe wear can also indicate how the horse places its feet. Very importantly, the feet are excellent indicators of where the horse might have some pain by how the feet compensate.

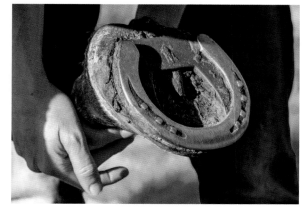

Conclude by carefully examining the foot for any signs of asymmetry. Assess the sole, the frog, ensure the heel has sufficient support, and inspect the shoe wear.

Your Palpation Findings and Manual Therapy Focus

You have completed your palpation examination and have your findings, which will be the focus of your manual therapy. You might be thinking about your management too and what you need to work on and change.

All muscles that are healthy and pliable can be massaged. However, you need to act cautiously in areas that are inflamed or damaged or where the horse is showing tenderness, as there could be an underlying injury that you should avoid. If the horse pulled away to your palpation in the upper neck for example, then you know that it is tender for it and will need some help, so you can try some of the more gentle techniques on that area to help the horse – even effleurage, which is a gentle technique you will learn, or some slow shaking. If you have chosen correctly, the horse will relax during the therapy and possibly close its eyes.

If the horse exhibits extreme tenderness, simply holding the area with a steady hand enables the horse to recognise that you acknowledge the site of pain. This is when you must stop and think about what you are doing and your management practices to cause this tension.

These are all reasons you palpate first before deciding on your therapy focus.

If the muscle is atrophied or firm to the touch and not very pliable, then you can go a little deeper into those tissues to promote better circulation, and if you feel an adhesion that feels like a tight band of tissue or a knot, you can go deeper to try to help it release. The horse, however, and its reactions, are always your guide to adjust pressure, to continue or to stop.

Evaluating Pain and Dysfunction in Your Horse

By now, you will be clear that many horses do have pain and dysfunction in their bodies, confirmed by your palpation findings, of which several contributory factors may be directly accountable to your management. These can produce discomfort and bring performance changes, behavioural changes and even changes in the horse's appearance.

Other factors can be a by-product of management – for example, issues you inherited when you acquired the horse, or the aging process. The root cause of pain and dysfunction can be challenging for horse owners and professionals to find, and often is caused by several factors, not just one. Identifying the numerous factors involves a systematic elimination process before you can help the horse. We know that physical, emotional and environmental influences play a big part in the overall health and wellbeing of the horse, as examined in Chapter 1. When something is not right with the horse, it can be due to a combination of failings in each or all of these areas. To help you to identify what might be causing pain and dysfunction in your horse, I will highlight specific areas for your focus in the checklists I have created further in this chapter.

COMPENSATIONS

When a horse has pain and dysfunction, it can cause it to compensate in other areas of its body, as it is unable to use the primary area effectively due to pain and discomfort from tension, impact (rubbing tack), farriery or dental inaccuracies, repetitive strain, over-training to one side of the body and so on. Therefore, it is far better that you find the primary dysfunction before compensatory patterns have become embedded in the horse. Eventually, this will lead to a breakdown in your horse in many areas, including the primary and the compensatory.

To avoid compensation, it is better to improve your management of the horse, treat it as an individual, recognise and understand its weakness so you can work with them, not expect too much of it, train it correctly and sympathetically, ensure tack fit and other management aspects, including its musculoskeletal system are ideal, so the horse has the best chance to stay sound in body and mind. I have intentionally emphasised the importance of this several times in this book.

ADAPTATIONS

When the horse's body has altered structurally, metabolically or neurologically, its body and mind must adapt in terms of movement and performance. Examples include bone fractures, nerve damage, injuries that have not repaired fully, limb amputation and loss of an eye, which causes the horse to move in a different way because the horse has no choice but to adapt if you require the horse to be in work and compete. This is different to when compensation occurs due to pain and dysfunction.

Your management is critical – especially regarding the horse's training and rest periods and your manual therapy focus so the horse's body can accept its adaptation and work with it. Precise treatment to support the horse is needed and will be enhanced by the right professional, whether a musculoskeletal therapist or a riding instructor or both. No force whatsoever should be used with an adaptation, as the body might not be able to react positively, so certain training aids might be unnecessary to avoid causing dysfunction. An empathic owner in these situations is essential and must never expect too much of the horse or too quickly. Adaptation can take a long time for the horse to accept.

OTHER BODY CONSIDERATIONS

These can have a definite impact on pain and dysfunction in a working horse and can cause gait compensations, including but not limited to:

- Conformation weakness when a length of bone and angles means the body cannot achieve specific movements comfortably.
- Bone conditions such as fractures, growth plate inflammation, chips, sore shins, abnormal bones in the feet (more common than we think), and joint, cartilage and ligament damage.
- Muscle conditions such as inflammation, tension and spasms causing restrictions in movement, adhesions and trigger points. Muscle atrophy which cannot support the correct movement of the skeleton, tendon and nerve damage.
- Internal features of the horse's body, such as an organ that might not function correctly, kidney, liver, stomach, colon, ovaries, testes and so on, necessitating a veterinary examination. Also its feed and nutrition.
- Dynamic features of a horse and knowing how to correctly assess the horse to ascertain if it is presenting with any unsoundness.

You might need professional assistance, and the key is knowing when to contact another professional for support or, if you suspect an underlying condition, a diagnosis by a veterinarian. Unfortunately, many horse owners leave it too long. When they receive help or a diagnosis of the condition, it is at an advanced stage and more difficult to address.

MULTIPLE FACTORS

Pain is usually a result of multiple factors or causes that contribute to a particular pain that the horse might exhibit in all three most common categories of performance, behaviour and appearance or only one. Generally, with horses, the pain is not attributed to a single cause but rather a result of a complex interplay between multiple factors.

For example, I might be called to a horse that is not working through its back comfortably; I might find that the original cause was a pain in its foot that has gone untreated, eventually leading to pain in its back because of the compensatory pattern the horse has developed to help it to move with less pain. When the horse uses its back differently, the saddle might not sit as it once did; therefore, it needs to be assessed for comfort and likely adjustment. This is where a chain reaction occurs with multiple causation factors. Another example might be a more straightforward solution whereby a horse presents with abdominal discomfort, and when I assess its diet, I usually find it is being overfed with too much concentrated feed and supplements, which is very common. When the horse is taken back to basics with a simpler forage and higher fibre-based diet with some additional vitamins and minerals if required, the horse's abdominal discomfort disappears, and its performance is regained.

These are the reasons we train our musculoskeletal therapists in my training school to the highest of standards, with life-long learning through their continuing professional development (CPD) training because they need the tools to work through a process of elimination and provide the right therapy. Unfortunately, many owners are very conscious of budget and expect us to offer a quick fix when it is anything but, especially if the presenting signs have been overlooked for some time. This is why I am dedicated to helping horse owners provide manual therapy on their own horses so they can maintain them between professional visits.

Checklists

To help you identify where and why your horse might be in pain, I have included some suggestions for you to consider in the form of checklists identifying the symptom and possible causes. These have been created within the common presenting categories in which pain has manifested and the possible causes.

The checklists are a structured, systematic method for identifying potential pain and causes, which help ensure that all relevant factors are considered. Many suggested reasons are repeated across the various presenting signs in all three checklists.

Working through the checklists reduces the likelihood of overlooking important details or making assumptions that could lead to inaccurate conclusions. Instead, you have an adequate basis for action

and collaboration, allowing multiple individuals to work together to identify the source of the pain, develop an effective solution and eliminate or reduce it.

CHANGE IN PERFORMANCE

A change in a horse's performance should always be investigated because it can be a sign of underlying health issues or other factors that could cause pain and impact the horse's well-being and ability to perform. For example, you might notice your horse not moving correctly, favouring a limb, reluctance to weight a limb, slower competition times, refusals to jump or navigate obstacles, difficulty maintaining pace and altered posture and gait.

Performance changes manifest in various ways, including decreased energy or enthusiasm, a decline in athletic ability or changes in behaviour while being ridden or handled. These changes may be due to various factors, such as lameness or joint problems, dental issues, gastrointestinal disorders, respiratory problems, poor nutrition, rider error and tack fit.

CHANGE IN BEHAVIOUR

It is necessary to investigate changes in a horse's behaviour, as it can often indicate underlying pain or discomfort that requires immediate attention. For instance, if your horse seems irritable, aggressive, less active than usual, has altered eating habits or displays avoidance behaviours such as avoiding being tacked or coming in from the field, it could be a sign of physical or psychological issues such as illness, injury, dental problems, gastrointestinal disorders, or stress. Ignoring changes in behaviour can lead to further health problems or exacerbate existing ones, potentially compromising the horse's welfare.

It is important to recognise and act upon these signs since horses communicate through gestures, as we know they cannot speak. When changes in behaviour are left unaddressed, the behaviour will worsen until the horse is labelled as dangerous, when it is merely trying to communicate its problem.

Horses are known to have headaches and other pain sources that can result in changes in behaviour.

CHANGE IN APPEARANCE

A change in appearance can also indicate pain, because it can be a sign of underlying health issues. Changes in a horse's appearance can manifest in various ways, including changes in weight or body condition, coat condition or the presence of lumps or bumps on the skin. These changes may be due to a wide range of factors, such as poor nutrition, skin conditions, parasites, allergies or underlying illness or injury. Investigation

and an appropriate treatment plan can help prevent a more serious health condition and more pain from occurring. Remember, in Chapter 4, the facial expressions that indicate pain.

By investigating changes in performance, behaviour and appearance, you can identify the underlying cause of the pain or problem and develop an appropriate treatment plan to address the issue. This can help prevent serious health problems, improve the horse's quality of life, and maintain its value and usefulness. Additionally, early detection and treatment of any issues can help to prevent accidents or injuries to both the horse and rider and possibly longer-term veterinary bills.

CHECKLIST RESULTS

Assuming you have the results after reviewing the checklists and are now ready to act and work through the likely causes…. This may involve looking at yourself and whether you are the cause through your actions or consulting with other healthcare professionals so you can obtain a definitive cause or diagnosis. Make sure you address all those points highlighted on your checklist, as what you think is a minor issue could be a huge contributing factor to pain. Depending on the specific cause of the pain, treatment may involve medication, adjusting training or riding programmes, changing the horse's living environment, providing manual therapy, changes in diet or management practices, change of tack, or other interventions.

Commit to a timeframe when working through the possible causes, and whilst you are doing this, avoid making the pain worse. For example, if you suspect the tack needs to be assessed, do not ride the horse. If you suspect the horse needs dental attention, arrange this immediately. If you put it off, the pain can worsen very quickly.

★ CHECKLIST

INDICATORS OF PAIN AFFECTING PERFORMANCE AND POSSIBLE CAUSES

1. Altered head carriage – dental, feet, bit/bridle, saddle/girth, training aids, horse on the forehand, rider error (rigid hands/asymmetry), emotional, physical injury, muscular.

2. Bit avoidance – bit/bridle, rider error (rigid hands), dental, feet, muscular.

3. Breathing changes/difficulties (including flaring nostrils, heaving, coughing, wheezing) – exercise intolerance, the horse is too weak, ridden in too much flexion, which contracts the windpipe, ridden in hyperflexion, overtraining the horse for its fitness and ability, riding in sand which is very tiring, saddle/girth – too tight impinging on lungs, rider weight, respiratory disorder needing veterinarian attention.

4. Change in performing certain movements – muscular, incorrect training, stress, rider error (rigid hands/asymmetry), bit/bridle, riding surface, saddle/girth, dental, feet, nutrition, weakness, undiagnosed condition.

5. Disunited – poor balance, lack of strength, poor conformation, incorrect training.

6. Focus altered – overtraining and insufficient rest, turn out and horse interaction inadequate, undiagnosed condition, nutrition and water intake inadequate, rider error (incorrect signals), pain.

7. Front limb interference – feet, muscular, bit/bridle, saddle/girth.

8. Halts to a stop abruptly – muscular, feet, fear, incorrect training, rider error (incorrect signals).

9. Height difference in movement of limbs – conformation, lameness, muscular, tendon, degenerative, neurological, riding surface.

10. High head carriage and hollow back – dental, bit/bride, saddle/girth, stress, fear, muscular, rider error (rigid hands/ asymmetry/ incorrect signals).

11. Jumping faults (loss of agility, refusing, not lengthening back, knocking poles) – rider error (weight/asymmetry), saddle/girth, feet, dental, sacroiliac, muscular, conformation weakness.

12. Lameness – full assessment required to find root cause. Usually bone related if occurs on firm ground and muscular if occurs on soft ground. Feet, conformation, muscular, bone, tendon, ligament, bit/bridle, saddle/girth, riding surface.

13. Limbs not weight bearing evenly (by imprints in the ground or sound of hooves) – lameness, feet, neurological, conformation, muscular, degenerative.

14. Mobility change – age, injury, lameness, neurological, degenerative, nutrition, conformation.

15. Neck and poll flexion and extension difficult – bit/bridle, dental, rider error (rigid hands/ asymmetry), head fixed in place with training aids, hay net placement, sinus or respiratory, muscular, neck vertebrae or degeneration such as osteoarthritis.

16. Producing too much saliva/foam/sweat – overheating, overworking, stress, underlying illness, infection, too much riding in flexion.

17. Reluctance to work (deemed 'lazy') – underlying health condition, nutrition, incorrect training, lack of fitness for demands, mental fatigue.

18. Schooling difficulties in general (shortened stride, not tracking up, unable to perform lateral work etc) – bit/bridle, saddle/girth, dental, feet, rider error (asymmetry/weight/incorrect signals), incorrect training, riding surface, health issue such as gastric ulcers, bone, sacroiliac, vertebrae, limbs, muscular.

19. Stiffness (moving in stable, shorter strides when ridden, movement not fluid) – joint, muscular, arthritis, bone infection, saddle/girth, incorrect training, lack of warm-up and cool-down, rider error (technique).

20. Stumbling, tripping, toe dragging – riding surface, fatigue, lameness, feet, joints, muscular, neurological, rider error (asymmetry/technique).

21. Tail swishing (in movement and between transitions or held to one side) – muscular, saddle/girth, undiagnosed condition, irritation, frustration/confusion with rider cues.

22. Tires more quickly – incorrect training, undiagnosed condition, nutrition, dehydration, age, environment (heat), bit/bridle, saddle/girth, rider error (weight).

23. Unable to work in collection and maintain – feet, dental, muscular, bit/bridle, saddle/girth, rider error (asymmetry/technique/signals), not on the bit, conformation, sacroiliac.

24. Unable to lengthen/stretch in exercise – bit/bridle, saddle/girth, rider error (asymmetry/weight/technique), muscular, gastrointestinal, sacroiliac.

25. Unable to maintain leads and track up – bit/bridle, saddle/girth, rider error (signals/asymmetry/weight), sacroiliac, muscular, training incorrect.

★ CHECKLIST

INDICATORS OF PAIN AFFECTING BEHAVIOUR AND POSSIBLE CAUSES

1. Aggressive towards other animals or people – fear, hormonal, undiagnosed condition, inadequate interaction/socialisation, poor handling/training practices.

2. Bucking, rearing, bunny-hopping gait, bolting – undiagnosed condition, sacroiliac, muscular, bit/bridle, girth/saddle, ridder error (rigid hands/tecnique/signals/asymmetry)

3. Cold backed (dipping back when mounted) – muscular, saddle/girth, rider error (technique/weight).

4. Girthy – gastric or hindgut ulcers, saddle/ girth, over-tightening of girth, girth galls, respiratory condition, muscular.

5. Grinding teeth – undiagnosed condition, stress, anxiety, frustration, hunger, dental, vice (a coping mechanism to a problem).

6. Head/ear shy – bit/bridle, ear mites, ear infection, sinus infection, knock to the head, previous ill-treatment such as twitching of ears, pain associated with past bad experiences.

7. Lying down more frequently – illness, injury, feet, muscular, aging/stamina.

8. Pawing at the ground – undiagnosed condition, muscular, hunger, thirst, anxiety, stress, boredom, the horse's needs are not being met.

9. Pointing of a limb, rubbing body parts, looking at flanks – the presence of pain at the location, gastric discomfort.

10. Resting body parts on equipment in stable (hay net, water feeder, resting hind feet on bedding banks) – sacroiliac pain, gastrointestinal, undiagnosed condition, feet.

11. Restlessness, agitation – undiagnosed condition, hunger or thirst, anxiety, stress, environment, lack of stimulation/interaction.

12. Rushing off when being mounted – muscular, saddle/girth, rider error (technique/weight), lack of training, fear, anxiety.

13. Sensitive to grooming, being tacked or rugged – muscular, injury, skin irritation, improper tack fit, sensory issue (more sensitive), digestive discomfort.

14. Spooking or shying – fear, anxiety, incorrect training, lack of exposure, rider error (handling/technique), vision/hearing problems.

15. Straining to urinate or defecate – undiagnosed condition, injury, muscular, sheath cleaning required, urinary/bladder issue, gastrointestinal.

16. Tail holding to one side or clamping – muscular/bone related, clamping tail often associated with gastrointestinal pain.

17. Turning away when a rider approaches horse with tack – incorrect training, discomfort from the rider, bit/bridle, saddle/girth.

18. Stereotypies (crib-biting, wind-sucking, weaving, box walking) – an environment not adequate or meeting horse's needs, lack of stimulation/interaction, gastrointestinal such as gastric ulcers, dental, undiagnosed condition, stress, anxiety, frustration.

19. Vocalising (groaning) – dental, gastrointestinal, muscular, bone, undiagnosed health condition, respiratory.

★ CHECKLIST

INDICATORS OF PAIN AFFECTING APPEARANCE AND POSSIBLE CAUSES

1. Condition – lacklustre, weight changes, abnormal swellings – nutrition, water intake, overworking and not enough rest, undiagnosed conditions, muscular, bone, hygiene, age, environment not adequate, neglect.

2. Discharge – eye or nasal that is not clear or odourless – infection, allergy.

3. Facial expressions/grimaces (generally exist and might be seen when exercised), muscular, bone, rider error (weight/asymmetry), bit/bridle, saddle/girth, incorrect training, respiratory, gastrointestinal.

4. Foot asymmetry (high heel/low heel, uneven hoof growth or shoe wear) – feet usually need remedial farriery, muscular, conformation not managed correctly.

5. Injury (cuts, abrasions, blood loss, swellings) – environment, incorrect training, or tack.

6. Muscle asymmetry, atrophy, hypertonicity – incorrect training, rider error (asymmetry), bit/bridle, saddle/girth, undiagnosed condition, injury not rehabilitated correctly or fully or re-injury has occured.

7. Skin (dull, dry, itchy, lumps, bumps) – management practice/cleanliness inadequate, nutrition, water, environmental allergy, tack cleanliness, undiagnosed condition.

8. Sweat patches (random patches for no apparent reason) – undiagnosed condition in region of sweat patch, usually an internal issue.

9. Tack areas (rub marks, white hairs, dry or broken skin, abrasions) – all tack needs addressing for suitability and fit and cleanliness of tack and horse.

10. Teeth (asymmetry, foul smell, quidding) – dental.

11. Tongue (cuts, abrasions, twisted) – dental, bit/bridle. Check bit is not broken. Rider error (rigid hands), training aids.

12. Posture changes (front limbs held close together, hind limbs held wide apart, hocks pointing inward, front limb pointing forward, hind limb pointing forward or further back) - undiagnosed condition, feet, nutrition, possible gastrointestinal, conformation not managed correctly.

13. Offloading weight from limbs when standing, weight shifting regularly – undiagnosed condition, joint pain, bone pain, arthritis, muscular, conformation.

14. Head position held differently (either lower or higher than usual or to the side) – bone, muscular, dental, bit/bridle, rider error (rigid hands), incorrect use of training aids blocking head/neck.

15. Rigid stance – undiagnosed condition.

16. Toes pointing in or out – foot, bone, joint, conformation.

17. Unable to stand comfortably with all four limbs perpendicular to the ground – undiagnosed condition, joint, bone, muscular, gastrointestinal.

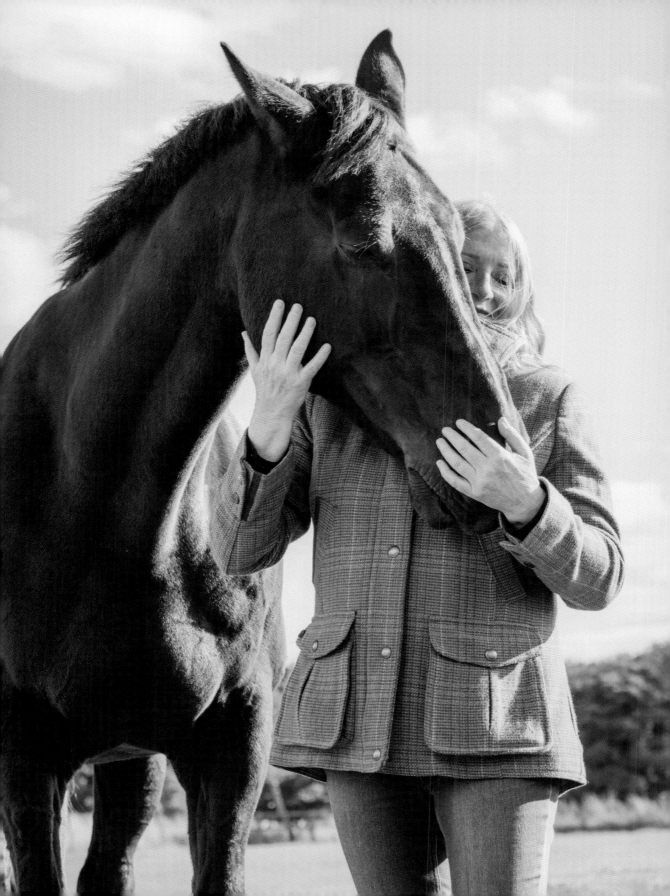

CHAPTER 7

Manual Therapy in Practice

It is important not to leap ahead to this chapter before completing the previous chapters, because a solid understanding and theoretical foundation are essential to ensure the safe and effective application of equine manual therapy. Also, you might be required to make some management changes that, combined with manual therapy, will maximise its benefits. It is a bespoke therapy you will provide for your horse depending on its needs, current state of health and the palpation examination, all covered in previous chapters.

By taking the time to understand the concepts behind equine manual therapy fully, you can ensure that you are using the correct techniques and adapting your approach to suit the individual needs of your horse. This will ultimately lead to better outcomes for the horse and a more rewarding and fulfilling experience for you.

Performing the Manual Therapy

Your horse will always be your guide when performing manual therapy; if it moves away in discomfort, either reduce your pressure, try another technique instead or stop altogether and move to another area. Nothing is achieved when the horse is uncomfortable or stands rigid during a manual therapy session, as muscle tissue can become inflamed or bruised if the horse is working against you.

Your intention is to work with the horse so it relaxes and enjoys the therapeutic experience by offering its body and mind to you. This will be indicated such as the horse pushing its body into your hands, sighing, closing its eyes, breathing more deeply, yawning and any other signs of relaxation it may display, which confirms the parasympathetic response is activated.

Perform manual therapy on both sides of the horse to ensure it feels balanced but work on one side first, complete that and then move on to the other. I usually start on the left side because the horse is used to most things starting there.

If the horse appears to be enjoying the manual therapy, you can continue, but if it is uncomfortable for the horse, you must stop to avoid bruising.

UNLEASHING THE HEALING POTENTIAL OF YOUR NEW SKILL

Equine manual therapy is a valuable tool for promoting the health and well-being of your horse. By following my tuition in this chapter, you can provide your horse with the benefits of regular manual therapy. Whether you want to improve your horse's performance, alleviate muscle soreness or simply bond with your equine companion, equine manual therapy can help you achieve your goals.

As you embark on your journey, remember to approach your horse with patience, sensitivity and respect. Listen to your horse's body language and adjust your technique accordingly. Take the time to develop a deep understanding of your horse's individual needs and preferences, and tailor your therapy sessions accordingly.

Above all, do not be afraid to experiment and explore. Equine manual therapy is both an art and a science, and every horse is unique. By embracing your own creativity and intuition, you can develop your own style and approach to manual therapy and help your horse achieve optimal health and happiness.

I sincerely hope the images and explanations in this chapter will give you the tools and inspiration you need to succeed. May you and your horse enjoy many happy and healthy years together with the help of the healing power of equine manual therapy.

Manual Therapy Techniques

Following on from explanations in Chapter 5:

MYOFASCIAL RELEASE

What? Myofascial release is a type of manual therapy that aims to release restricted fascia, tension and pain in the body; it is a layer of connective tissue that surrounds muscles, bones and organs. Myofascial release can stimulate the release of endorphins, which are natural pain-relieving chemicals produced by the body. Endorphins can promote a sense of relaxation and well-being, which can further enhance the relaxing effects of myofascial release.

Where? Myofascial release can be applied to any part of the horse's body because fascia is everywhere beneath the horse's skin. Fascia should feel pliable and elastic on palpation. The fascia that feels stuck or moves slowly under your hand will need a release. You might also find an area where there is a trigger point in the fascia, where it originates, and the horse will flinch on palpation, or the trigger point might be elsewhere because trigger points can cause referred pain to another part of the horse's body. A trigger point is a sensitive spot in the fascia or muscle.

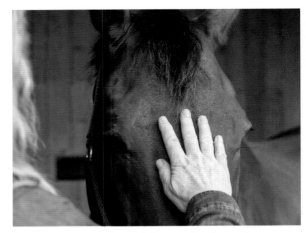

Slide your open palm and fingers slowly up the centre of the forehead to the base of the forelock. If you feel a barrier or a restriction in the tissue or it slows down under your fingers, remain static on that area for a few moments before continuing.

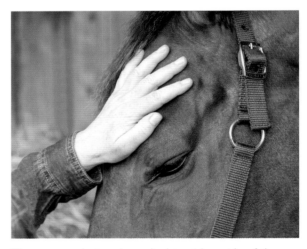

The same technique is applied to either side of the forehead muscles to the base of the ear, to the right and then to the left. This horse finds myofascial release work very relaxing, as you can see from his expression.

Myofascial release works with a broader network of restrictions throughout the horse's body.

When? Because myofascial release has many benefits, it is a therapy that can be applied at any time to the horse. It can be applied gently in a sports massage (pre-competition) but is very beneficial in maintenance and remedial treatments because it helps to relax the horse.

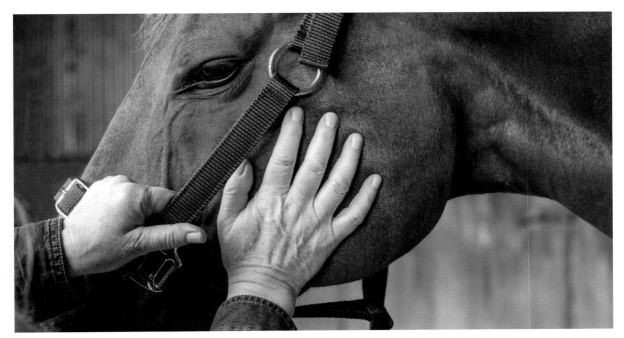

Use the palm of the hand and fingers to connect with the fascia in the masseter muscles (cheek). Starting at the lower edge, slowly upward, following the curve of the cheek engaging the fascia with your hand and fingers, sweeping around the entire mandible (jaw).

How? Very slowly, pressure is applied to the horse's body with hands either with a single-hand or double-handed with the flat of the hand or by gently clenching the fist and using the flat finger area between the knuckles. The intention is to engage with the superficial fascia (beneath the skin) and then release it by performing a slow, stretching-type movement with light to moderate pressure. It can be performed multiple times over the same area to release large bands of restricted fascia. The tissue is worked until a release is felt and becomes more elastic and pliable. This may occur in one session, but it may require multiple sessions depending on how long the fascia has been restricted.

Myofascial Release to Forehead

Myofascial release to the forehead is similar to the palpation; just a little more engagement with the tissue is needed, but this area of fascia is thin because it is covering mostly bone. If the horse reacts negatively, gently stay on the area with a steady hand until it gets used to you being there.

Myofascial Release to Cheeks

Very similar to the palpation, but you are engaging with the fascia and working with it, and if you find any restrictions in the tissue, hold for a few moments. It might release immediately, but it might take a few attempts or in future sessions. Continue to perform

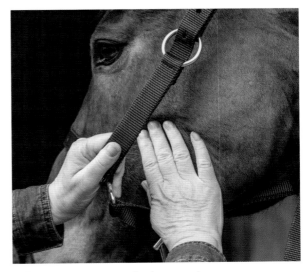

1. Starting position at the lower edge.

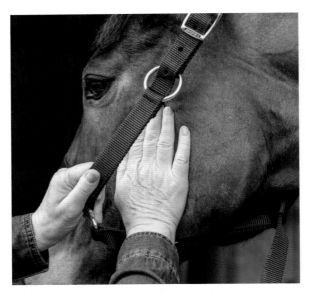

2 Next continue alongside the cheekbone.

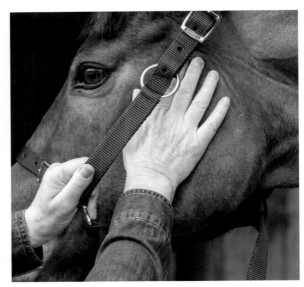

3. Approach the upper edge of the cheek.

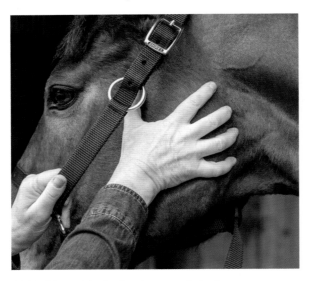

4. Working with the fascia around the jaw.

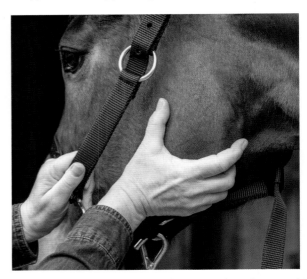

5. Encompassing the entirety of the horse's jawbone within your hand, actively connecting with the fascia, glide back to the starting position. Repeat the process as needed.

several times if the horse enjoys it. If the horse is sensitive, think about the likely causes.

To ensure you fully apply myofascial release to the cheek area, it is performed in a pattern.

Myofascial Release to the Neck

This technique can be performed using both hands descending along the horse's neck, with one hand following the other. Connect with the fascia and apply gentle traction to stretch the fascia throughout the entire neck. Alternatively, you can opt for a double-handed approach, which can provide a deeper release.

As you connect with the fascia, you may see a noticeable fold or indentation in the skin before your hands due to the fascia lying slightly deeper beneath

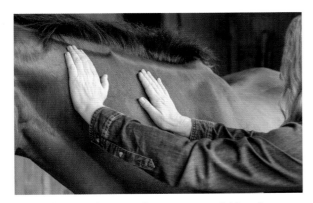

1. Myofascial release with two sequential hands.

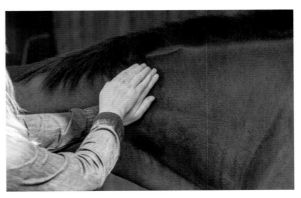

2. Myofascial release with double hands.

the surface of the skin. If you come across areas where you sense restrictions in the fascia or where the horse indicates it is beneficial, you can perform a static hold, maintaining gentle pressure. If needed, you can repeat this process up to three times.

Myofascial Release to Shoulder

The most effective way to perform this technique is by employing the double-handed flat knuckles method, which allows for the deepest engagement with the fascia.

The sequence begins at the withers and proceeds down the front edge of the shoulder, running parallel to the neck, until reaching the chest. Then, continue working down the central shoulder region, to the top of the forelimb. Finally, to the outer edge of the shoulder, adjacent to the back and ribs. Throughout the process, maintain a slow pace, actively engaging with the fascia. If you encounter any restrictions or areas that feel stuck, pause for a few moments as they may release before moving on. Make sure to cover the entire shoulder area thoroughly. Repeat this sequence up to three times if needed.

As you reach the final step of working on the outer edge of the shoulder, take advantage of addressing any heavily restricted fascia caused by the girth. Adjust your right hand closer to the girth region and continue the technique. It is likely that you will encounter fascial restrictions beneath your hand, which may produce a sensation sim-

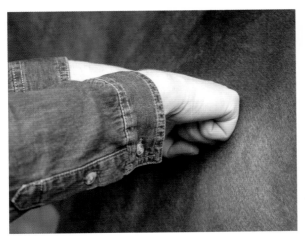

The double-handed flat knuckle hand position. Take care to glide the flat part of the fingers between the knuckles to avoid digging into the horse's tissues..

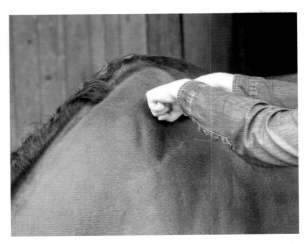

Demonstrating the starting point of the central shoulder region.

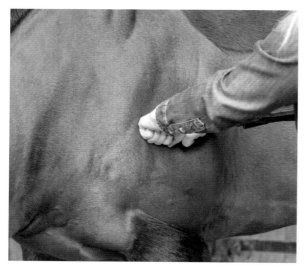

Continuing to descend the shoulder.

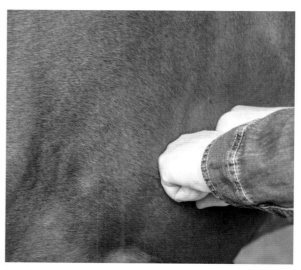

Reaching the lower edge of the central shoulder region.

ilar to the popping of bubble wrap. Be mindful of the horse's sensitivity in this area, so apply gentle pressure. Performing this step multiple times can be beneficial until you feel an improvement in the fascia and observe a positive response from the horse.

Myofascial Release to the Back and Ribs

There are various approaches to performing this, all centred around the core principle of releasing fascial restrictions where they feel stuck or exhibit slower movement under your hand. It is important to cover the entire back area, extending from the withers to

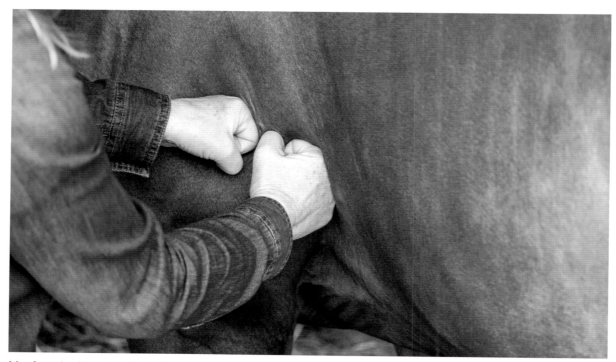

Myofascial release to the girth area.

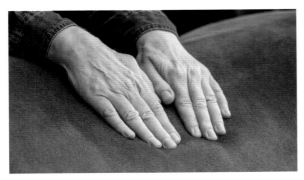

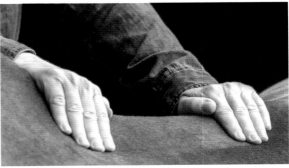

Standing on a secure platform so you can work into the back once the horse is comfortable with your position, start with hands side by side and engage with the fascia.

Slowly move one hand away as it stretches the fascia along the back away from the anchor hand. Repeat this action over the back until you approach the boundary where the ribs become noticeable. My right hand, positioned near the withers, remains stationary as the anchor hand, while the other hand acts as the working hand, progressing towards the lumbar region.

the lumbar region, located just behind the saddle and in front of the croup. Repeat the process up to three times if necessary, ensuring the horse remains comfortable throughout.

When working with horses experiencing a sore back, utilising the flat part of your hands can be highly beneficial. This technique allows for an effective release of fascia while minimising pressure on tender tissues.

Releasing fascia over a horse's ribs is beneficial, as it can help improve their breathing and overall respiratory function and fascial restrictions caused by the rider's leg position.

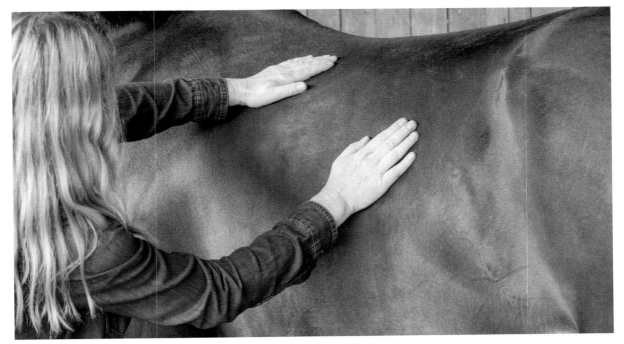

Stretching the fascia over the ribs, reducing your pressure applied in this area. Cover the entire area to the eighteenth rib in a manner that feels comfortable and effective to you.

Myofascial Release to the Hindquarters

Releasing fascia on the hindquarters of a horse typically requires slightly more pressure due to the substantial muscling and thickened fascia in this area. You can choose to apply the technique using double-handed flat knuckles, similar to what was done on the shoulder, or utilise the method of flat hands with an anchor hand and a working hand or with both hands placed on top of each other. Make sure to cover the entire hindquarters area thoroughly. Repeat the process up to three times if needed.

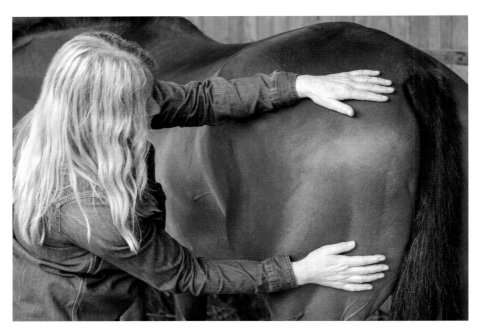

Establishing my left hand as the anchor, I use my right hand to stretch the fascia away from the anchor towards the lower hamstring area. Ensure the entire area is covered, finishing at the hock.

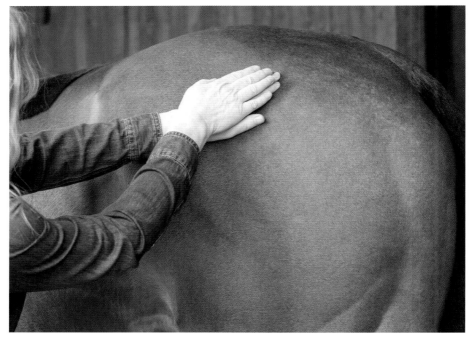

With two hands, this involves you engaging your body weight to provide the desired level of pressure and maintain a balanced and controlled application.

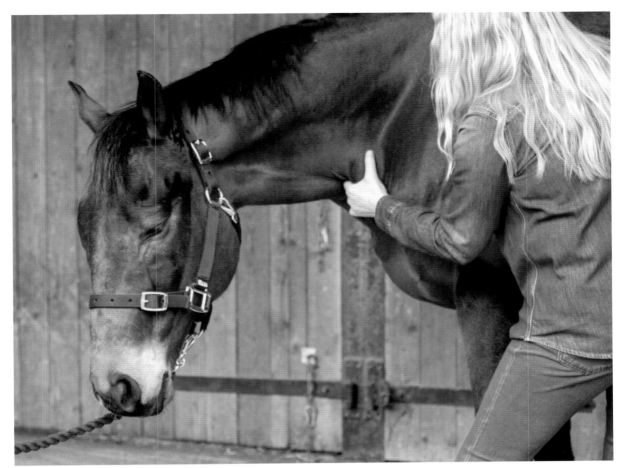

Once the muscle and fascia were loosened, I carefully positioned my hand around the precise area where the trigger point was identified and maintained a gentle hold. In response, the horse turned his head towards me, finding relief and closed its eyes. I maintained this therapeutic contact, holding the position for a few minutes until the horse naturally moved away, signifying the completion of the trigger point release.

Trigger Point Therapy – Bonus Technique

My intention in this book was not to provide detailed instruction on trigger point therapy, as it is challenging to convey accurately through images alone. However, while demonstrating the techniques on this horse, I unexpectedly discovered a tender trigger point in the cervical fascia. It was causing discomfort for the horse and eliciting a 'twitch response' across his shoulder. To address this, I began to soften the area using myofascial release, followed by the application of trigger point therapy.

TENSION POINT RELEASE (TPR)

What? TPR is a gentle manual therapy that targets specific tension points in a horse's body to release physical tension and address emotional issues. These tension points are located at specific junctions over bone. TPR allows the horse to release tension through gentle touch and can be considered as a form of energy healing, as it supports the body's natural healing abilities. Horses that have experienced significant changes, such as new owners, environments, training routines, rescue from abuse, or those with demanding training and competition schedules (for example, racehorses), can benefit from the subtle nature of TPR. Some horses, due to their background, may avoid human contact and touch, but they can still benefit from the non-invasive approach of TPR. Horses with specific personality traits, such as being stoic or closed off, who struggle to express themselves, may find a way to do so during this therapy. Additionally, anxious and tense horses with difficulty relaxing often respond well to TPR and experience profound releases.

Where? It is applied to specific identified common tension points throughout the horse's body over bone landmarks. You are not working directly with the muscles and fascia – instead you are working with tension that accumulates around crucial areas of the skeleton but which does affect neighbouring soft tissues.

When? Due to the nature of this gentle therapy, it can be applied anytime to the horse but has the most benefit when in a quiet environment. TPR can be periodic as a stand-alone treatment or incorporated into any manual therapy session; it can be applied at the beginning with an anxious horse, but it is very beneficial to finish with as a gentle way to close the session. If you find an area of the horse particularly sensitive during your manual therapy session, you can focus on that area at the end with a little TPR work.

How? Using the fingertips or the hand, apply a gentle contact of a very light touch to the horse. There is no real pressure involved. You simply place your fingers or hand on the horse just enough so it knows you are there. This is a simple, non-invasive, yet very powerful technique that horses respond well to. Once you complete one side of the horse, complete the opposite side to balance it. The horse may need to release on one point or several. Be very patient, it is a slow process.

Your intention is important in that you visualise the horse releasing its body tension as you are holding the point. Hold the position for a few moments, between twenty seconds to two minutes, depending on the horse's reactions and acceptance. If the horse starts to release, stay on the point. Then, once the horse has indicated its release by the relaxing signs it is giving, wait until it moves, then step back and allow it a moment before moving on to the next point. This applies to all points.

Point one – this is the position indicated by the thumb in front of the eye and fingers below, partly resting on the cheekbone.

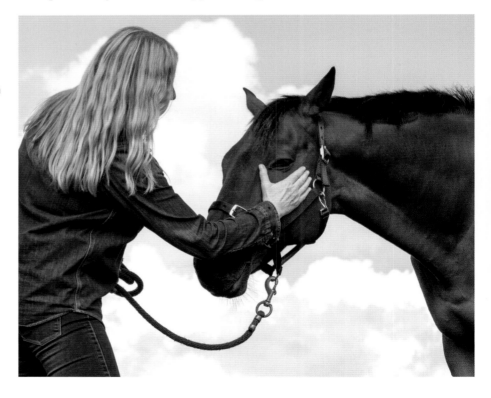

Point two – located at the hinge of the TMJ. The image shows the horse's eyes closing whilst in the process of a release.

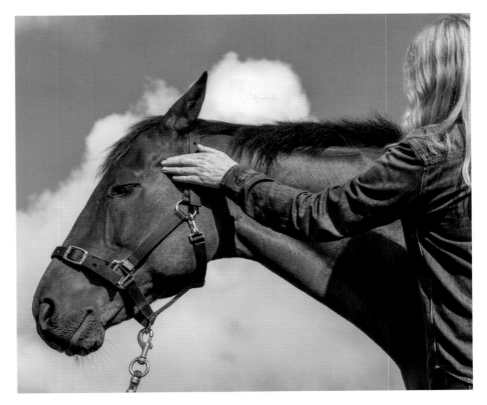

Point three – located in the upper cervical region, about one hand width behind the ears. The horse has heavy eyes and has lowered his head whilst in the process of a release.

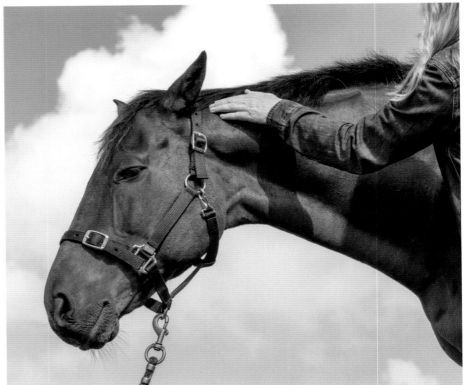

Point four – located at the base of the neck, midway between the top and lower edge of the inside shoulder.

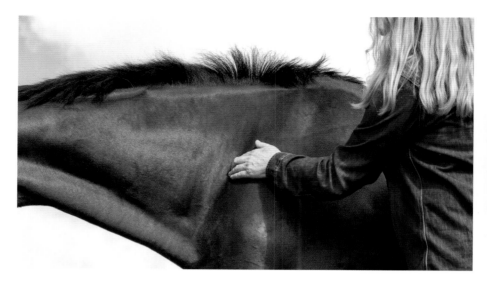

Point five – located on the horse's point of shoulder, the bone prominence at the edge of the humerus, where it meets the scapula.

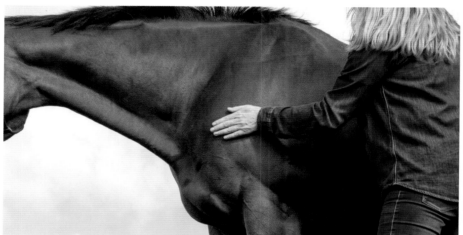

Point six – located on the horse's ribs in the girth area; behind this point is the horse's heart.

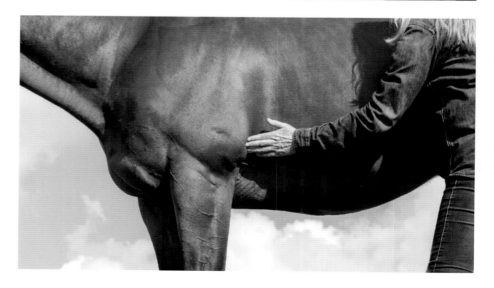

Point seven – located on the withers, at around thoracic three. The point is held with a thumb on the left side and an index or second finger on the right. Sometimes you may need to move your position further forward on the withers or further back to locate the exact point for your horse.

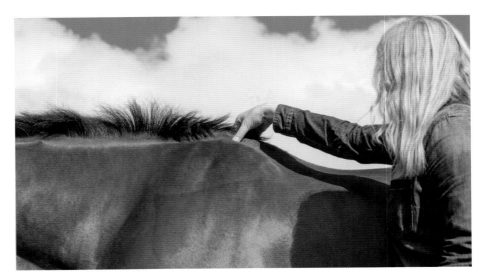

Point eight – located mid-back at around thoracic fourteen. There are eighteen thoracic vertebrae in total in most horses, so you can count back from the last rib and then move your hand up onto the thoracic vertebrae to find the point.

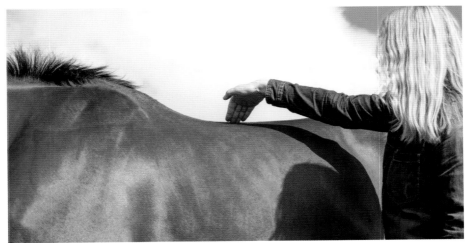

Point nine – the point of the tuber sacrale or croup. Place three fingers over the bone prominence. You can place either side on the bone or in the centre.

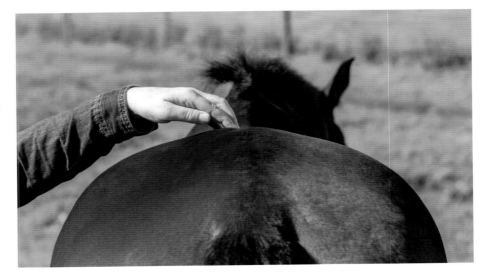

Point ten – located on the sacrum in front of the tail, the point requires the flat of the hand to lie over the sacrum.

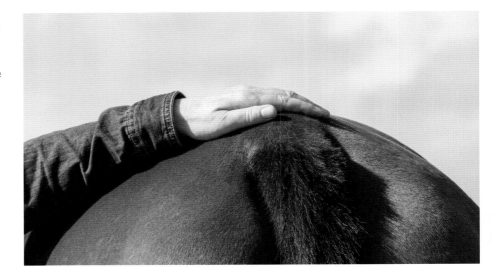

Point eleven – located on the tuber coxa (false hip bone). Place three fingers on top of the bone.

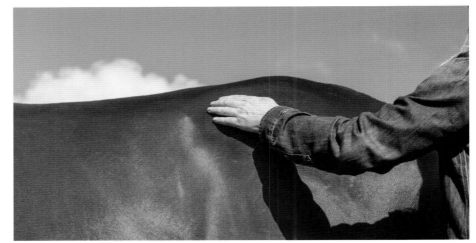

Point twelve – located over the stifle. The hand is placed flat on the muscling to cover the entire point.

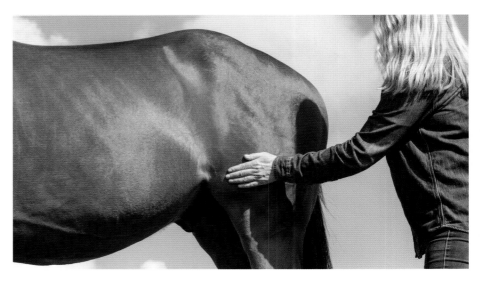

Point thirteen – this is almost midway down the hamstring muscling, the flat hand is placed over the entire point, and underneath lies the ischium, the horse's seat bone.

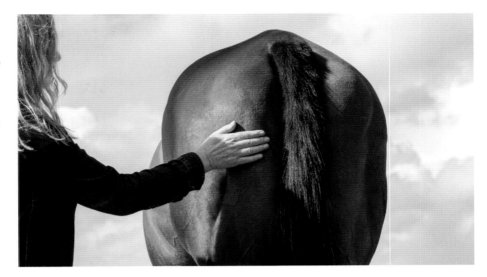

Point fourteen – located on the carpus (knee). Place the flat of one hand on the front and the other on the back of the carpus.

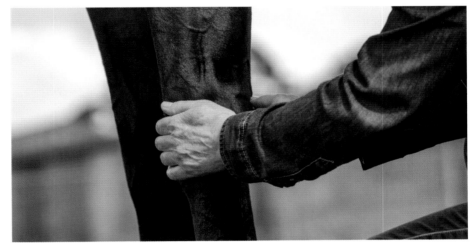

Point fifteen – located on tarsus (hock). Place one hand around the hock, this position often requires you to move slightly depending on the horse's needs. The other hand is free, but if you know your horse well and there is no risk of kicking out, both hands can be placed around the tarsus.

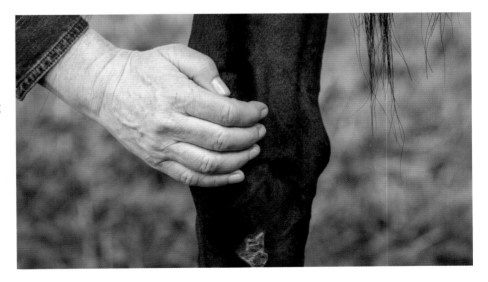

EFFLEURAGE

What? Effleurage is a massage technique that involves long, gliding strokes. The term 'effleurage' originates from the French word *effleurer*, which means 'to skim' or 'to touch lightly'. It is commonly used to help stimulate circulation, reduce muscle tension, and promote relaxation because, when performed slowly, it has a very calming effect. The technique involves using light to moderate pressure of gliding strokes over the horse's body towards the lymph nodes distributed throughout the body and connected to the lymphatic vessels. Effleurage helps stimulate the lymphatic system and improves its functioning by removing toxins from the body.

Where? It can be performed all over the horse's body by following the direction of the coat towards the lymph nodes within the horse's circulatory system. For this purpose, the effleurage gliding technique is aimed at the horse's chest, its elbow/heart area, the groin/stifle and just inside the back legs toward the hock.

- **Region one** – gliding down the neck, over the front of the shoulder, towards the lymph nodes in the chest area just inside the forelimb.
- **Region two** – gliding over the entire shoulder, towards the lymph nodes in the chest just inside the forelimb or those in the elbow/heart area.
- **Region three** – gliding over the back and ribs, towards the lymph nodes in the groin/stifle area.
- **Region four** – gliding over the hindquarters, towards the lymph nodes inside the hindlimbs, towards the hock.

When? After the initial palpation, effleurage is your first conversation with the horse's body for manual therapy; it allows the horse to truly engage with the sensation of your hands as you start. It is often used at the start and end of the treatment to warm up the muscles and relax the horse, for around five minutes and at the end for five minutes to help expel toxins.

This technique is most beneficial within the

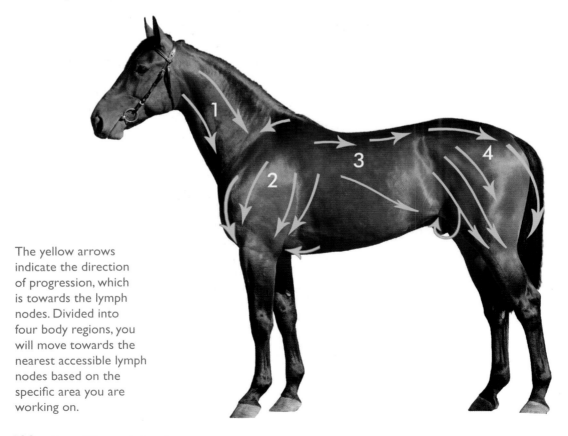

The yellow arrows indicate the direction of progression, which is towards the lymph nodes. Divided into four body regions, you will move towards the nearest accessible lymph nodes based on the specific area you are working on.

sub-categories of: sports (pre-competition and post-competition), maintenance and remedial.

How? The hands mould to the shape of the body part in a smooth, gliding movement, following the direction of the horse's coat. The rhythm is essential because a slow pace invokes relaxation through the parasympathetic nervous system response, while a quicker pace stimulates the horse. Most horses prefer a slow pace as it is very soothing, helping to relax tense muscles and promote a sense of calm and wellbeing.

The effleurage technique involves starting with a leading hand, and gently gliding it in the desired direction. As the leading hand completes its stroke, lift it off the horse and cross over the following hand. Repeat this process continuously, creating a smooth and uninterrupted flow that effortlessly glides over the contours of the horse, aiming towards the lymph nodes. This motion resembles a seamless wave-like motion.

Effleurage to the Neck

Follow the technique to cover the entire neck, always working towards the lymph nodes in the chest, just inside the forelimb. Repeat several times.

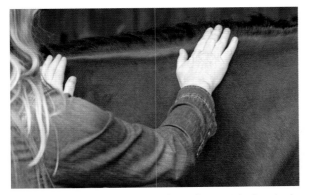

With both hands on the horse's neck, my right hand takes the lead, followed by the left. The right hand smoothly slides across the neck and descends in front of the shoulder, moving towards the lymph glands in the chest.

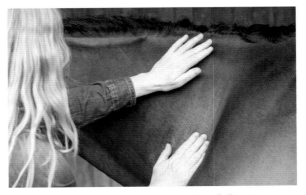

My left hand mimics the same motion, following the same path as it glides towards the front of the shoulder.

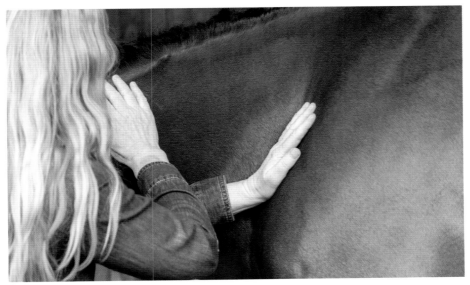

Lifting off from the horse, the right hand crosses the left and returns to the starting point on the neck, reclaiming its position as the leading hand. This repetitive pattern forms the wave-like motion that should be maintained.

Effleurage to the Shoulder

The technique is repeated over the shoulder, working towards the chest at the front of the shoulder inside the forelimb or the elbow/heart area at the rear of the shoulder, whichever is more comfortable for you. Complete effleurage over the entire shoulder from the withers to the forelimb. Repeat several times.

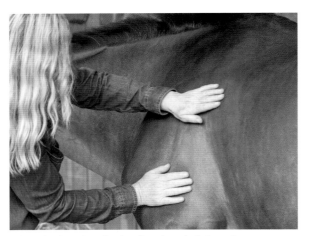

My right hand is the leading hand gliding down the entire shoulder with my left hand following.

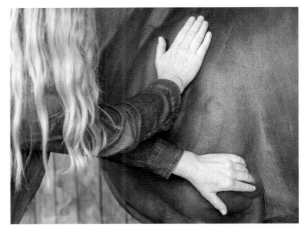

When my right hand completes its stroke, it crosses over the left and returns to start again.

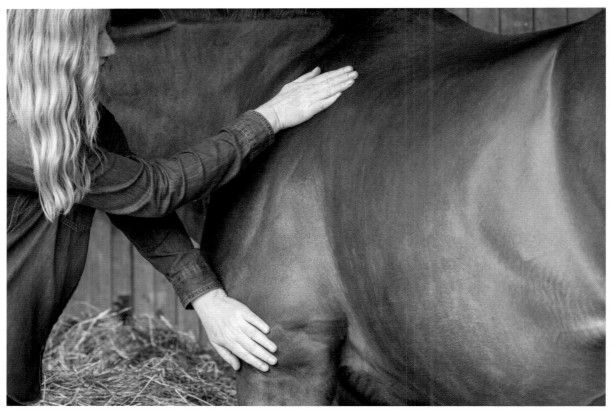

Cover the entire shoulder area by working with hands closer together or further apart, as shown here.

Effleurage to the Back and Ribs

Repeat the effleurage technique several times to ensure you cover the entire back from the withers to the lumbar muscles, including the entire rib cage region, always working towards the groin/stifle area.

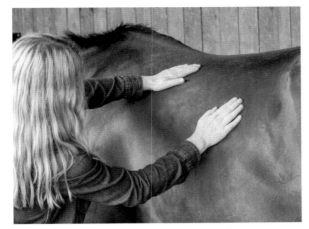

Starting on the back, with my right hand as the leading hand, followed by the left, covering the entire back.

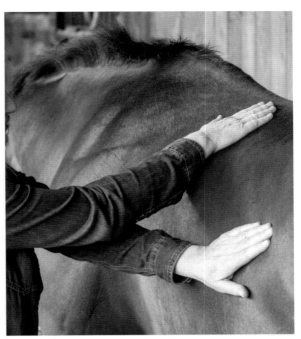

When each stroke is complete, the right hand crosses the left, and the sequence is repeated.

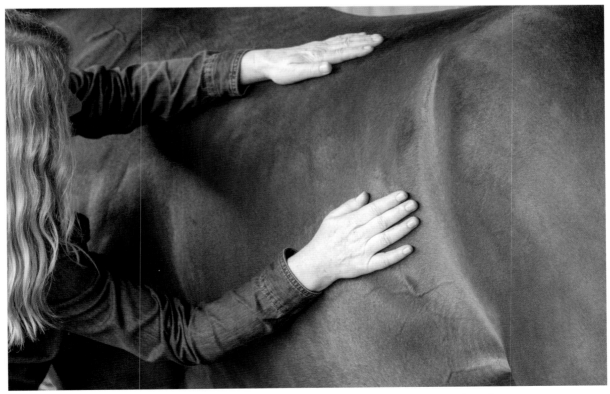

Working over the ribs, my right hand is gliding towards the groin/stifle area, to complete the sequence.

Effleurage to the Hindquarters

Perform the effleurage technique multiple times on the hindquarters, applying increased pressure com-pared to other body parts, considering the substantial muscling. Always work towards the inside of the hindlimbs, directing the movement towards the hock.

Encompassing the upper and middle sections of the hindquarters.

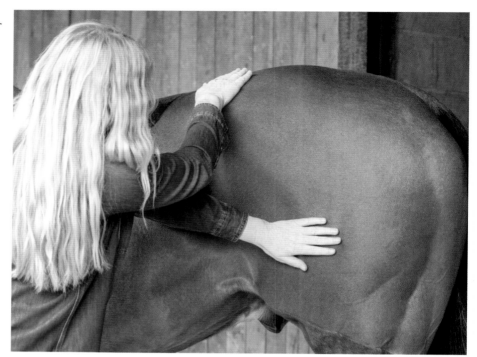

Working to the hamstring area, always adopting the same technique.

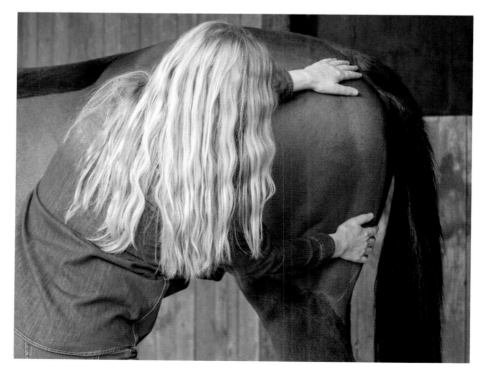

TAPOTEMENT

What? Tapotement originates from the French word that means 'tapping'. It is a massage technique with a more energising and stimulating effect, usually performed with light pressure for a short duration to increase circulation and can therefore be warming to the tissues. It can help break down fibrous adhesions in the tissues and penetrate the deeper muscles. It is a highly vibratory technique and three techniques are shown which make up the tapotement trio.

Where? The techniques in the tapotement category can be applied to the horse's shoulder, back and hindquarters, avoiding the neck as they are too stimulating.

If you have discovered the horse is tender on palpation, avoid tapotement in those areas, because already inflamed tissue could be exacerbated.

When? The main intention is to perform tapotement before the horse is worked, just enough to help the tissues to be more pliable, which can also help to reduce injury. It can also be useful to apply to the deeper muscles of the hindquarters. Tapotement would never be performed after the horse has worked, competed or is dehydrated and very rarely in a maintenance or remedial session unless the horse was very cold and needed to be quickly warmed. If performed too deeply or for too long, it can cause muscle fatigue, making the horse feel tired; as such, I recommend the maximum applications you should perform with tapotement in the relevant body part sections.

This is most beneficial within the sub-categories of: sports (pre-competition).

How? The tapotement trio comprises cupping, hacking and pounding, all of which are performed in their distinct style but always in a light, rhythmical manner with loose wrists and elbows.

CUPPING

The hands are cupped in a relaxed shape, keeping the fingers together, the fingertips and the heel of the hand touch the horse. Performed with alternative hands, rapid but light. A hollow clapping sound will be produced as the air is trapped between your hands on the horse's skin; this helps to stimulate the capillaries to bring blood to the surface.

Cupping can be applied to the horse's shoulder, the back and the hindquarters, always avoiding the neck.

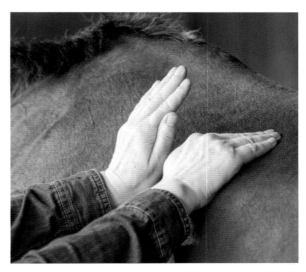

Demonstrating the two phases of the cupping technique. Right hand making contact with the horse first.

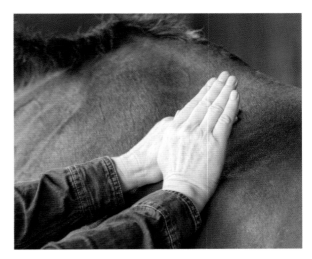

The hands exchange position to create the cupping technique as the left hand makes contact with the horse.

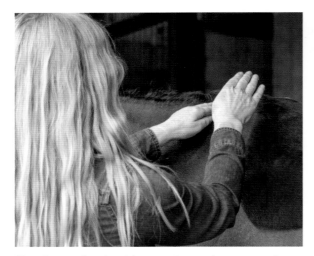

Cupping to the shoulder starting at the upper edge

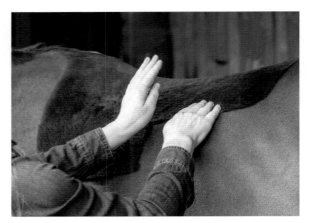

Cupping to the back all the way along. My right hand is at the lowest point, where it stops at the junction with the rib edge.

Cupping to the Shoulder

Proceed with the sequence by moving from left to right, slightly lowering and continuing from right to left. Repeat this pattern, dropping down slightly on the shoulder each time, as you move from left to right and right to left again. The objective is to ensure no area of the shoulder region is missed.

As you progress to the lower section of the shoulder, it is necessary to adjust your body positioning. Maintain a straight back, engage your core, open your legs and adopt a posture similar to a partial squat. Upon completing the entire sequence and reaching the lower edge of the shoulder, just above the fore-limb, return to the starting position and repeat the sequence. If needed, you can repeat the sequence for a maximum of three repetitions.

Cupping to the Back

Proceed with the sequence by starting at the withers and working down towards the rib edge, then slightly shifting to the right muscling and performing upward cupping towards the withers from the rib edge. Continue this pattern along the entire back, focusing on the muscling between the vertebrae and the rib edge. Once you reach the end of the back at the lumbar region, walk back to the starting point and repeat the sequence from left to right. You can repeat the sequence up to a maximum of three times.

Cupping to the Hindquarters

Continue the sequence by extending the technique to the top of the hindquarters (you may need to stand on a secure step), moving from left to right and right to left, similar to how you did on the shoulder. Then proceed to the middle section, from the tuber coxa around to the hamstrings, again moving from left to right and right to left, until you reach the lower edge of the hindquarters at the top of the hind leg.

To accommodate the lower section of the hindquarters, it is important to adjust your body positioning. Maintain a straight back, engage your core, open your legs and adopt a posture resembling a partial squat. Please note that performing this technique over the hindquarters can be tiring; if able, you can repeat the sequence up to a maximum of three times.

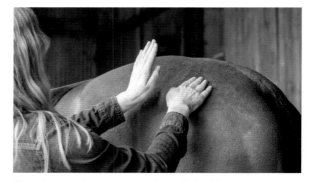

Cupping to the upper section of the hindquarters over the gluteal muscles.

HACKING

The edge of the hand makes contact with the horse's body in an alternative, rapid but light tapping movement. Hacking assists with the breakup of congestion in the muscle fibres and can be applied over the areas where cupping has been performed, the shoulder, the back and the hindquarters but again, always avoiding the neck.

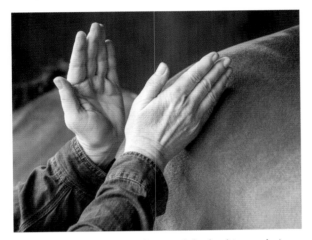

Demonstrating the two phases of the hacking technique. Right hand making contact with the horse first.

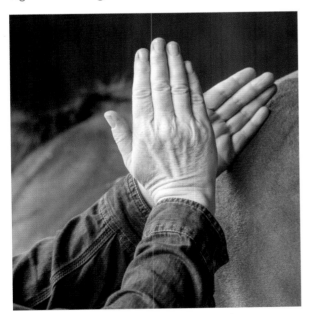

The hands exchange position to create the hacking technique as the left hand makes contact with the horse.

Hacking to the Shoulder, Back and Hindquarters

The sequence is applied the same as with 'cupping', and you can repeat this up to a maximum of three times over each body area.

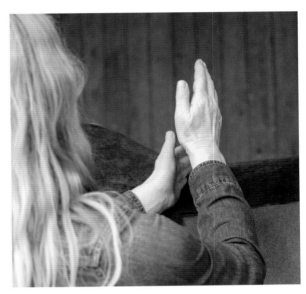

Hacking along the horse's back.

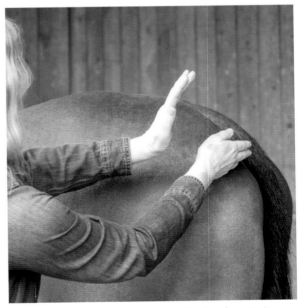

Hacking to the upper section of the hindquarters.

POUNDING

Pounding serves as the final technique in the tapotement trio. To perform this technique, create a loose fist with your hand, and make contact with the horse's body using the edge of the fist. Utilise a rapid, drumming-type movement with alternate hands similar to cupping and hacking. Pounding is specifically applied to the upper section of the horse's hindquarters, targeting the deeper muscles and promoting circulation in this heavily muscled area.

Exercise caution and avoid pounding over bony landmarks such as the tuber sacrale (croup) and tuber coxae (hip). Limit the application of this technique to a maximum of three repetitions. It is important not to apply pounding to the neck, shoulder or back regions.

Always conclude the tapotement trio of techniques with some effleurage to help expel any accumulated toxins.

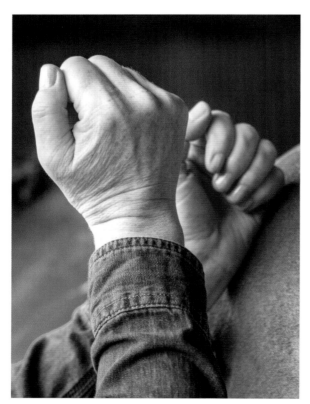

Demonstrating the pounding technique to the upper section of the hindquarters.

SHAKING

What? The term 'shaking' originates from the Latin word *vibrare*, which means 'to shake' or 'to vibrate'. This massage technique is a rhythmic shaking performed gently either single-handed, double-handed or with fingertips. It is used to stimulate the muscles and increase circulation, helping to loosen tissue to reduce tension and stiffness in the horse's body. It can be used as a prelude to other techniques that can be applied a little deeper, such as compression or myofascial release. Shaking slowly can also help improve nerve function and induce the parasympathetic nervous system to help the horse relax.

Where? Shaking can be performed slowly over the neck (single-handed), shoulder, back, abdomen and hindquarters (double-handed). You can also perform with your fingertips over and around bony landmarks to help loosen up the soft tissue attachments in the areas such as the point of the shoulder, the elbow region, along the spine, the tuber sacrale (croup), the tuber coxa (hip) and the dock of the tail, and also, gently over the knee, hock and fetlock. It can also help to reduce joint swelling if osteoarthritis is present. It is best to avoid the horse's face.

When? This technique can be performed at any time; it is very versatile. It is most beneficial within the sub-categories of: sports (pre-competition and post-competition), maintenance and remedial.

How? It is performed with the flat of the hand(s) by shaking the tissue from side to side or up and down over large muscular areas or with the fingertips around the bony prominences, as this is a higher frequency technique, as such it is more like a 'vibration'. Stay in a continuous contact with the horse whilst shaking, then lift off, move to the adjacent area, and perform again. You should feel the tissue slightly stretching as you complete the shake. Performing slowly will relax the horse, and performing rapidly can stimulate it.

Shaking can be applied to the neck single-handedly, to the shoulder double-handed (hands side by side), to the back double-handed and the same to the hindquarters; ensure you cover the hindquarters, as it is excellent for loosening the hamstring area.

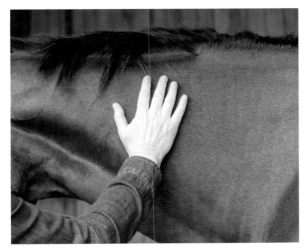

Shaking is applied single-handedly to the neck.

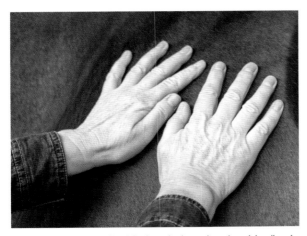

Shaking is applied double-handed to the shoulder/back.

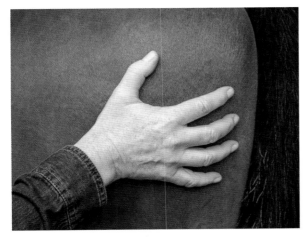

Shaking is applied to the hamstring area in the hindquarters.

COMPRESSION

What? The primary purpose of compression is vasodilation, which is a widening of the blood vessels to increase blood circulation. Compression helps relieve tense muscles by spreading the muscle fibres, promoting relaxation and pain relief. If the tissues are inflamed or tender, avoid those areas, as it could cause bruising.

Where? Compression is applied over larger muscle groups such as the crest of the neck (splenius m. and rhomboid m.), the lower side of the neck where it meets the shoulder single-handed (serratus ventralis m.), the lower half of the shoulder and forearm double-handed (triceps m.), the hip flexor muscles double-handed (tensor fascia lata m.), the hamstring group of muscles double-handed (semitendinosus m., etc.). Compression to all these areas on one side of the horse should take around ten minutes and twenty on both sides. Take more time in areas where the horse shows enjoyment or where you can feel tension or a change in tissue texture, indicating greater pliability.

When? This can be performed as part of a regular maintenance massage, such as a weekly session, or an occasional remedial massage. Both occasions would allow you to spend more time with this technique, as it can be applied in various styles and durations depending on the body region. Most beneficial within the sub-categories of maintenance and remedial.

How? Compression is performed by applying pressure to the area in a rhythmic circular motion clockwise and then gliding your hand(s) over to the adjacent tissue area and repeating the circular motion sequence. Whilst performing, the underlying tissue is moved. On large muscle groups such as the hindquarters, the pressure can be firmer, but you must be careful not to nip the horse or go too deep, as you may bruise the tissue. Always listen to the horse; if it moves away from the pressure, it is too deep. It can be performed to larger areas with a loosely clenched fist using the flat part of the fingers between the knuckles, known as single-handed compression, or by using both hands, known as double-handed compression. Compression can be applied to smaller areas of the body with the fingertips.

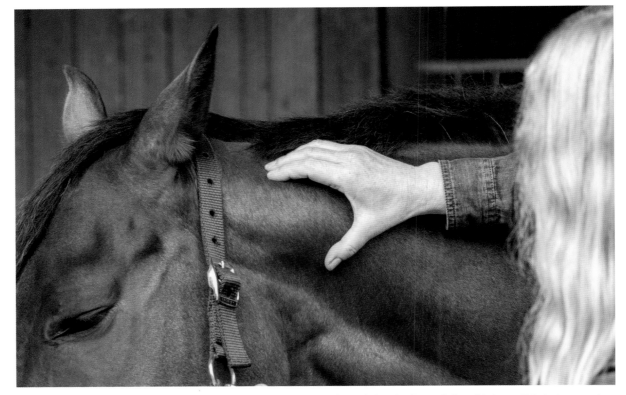

Fingertip compression is applied to the upper cervical muscles whilst the horse's head is in a slightly lowered position. The horse is indicating complete relaxation with his eyes closed.

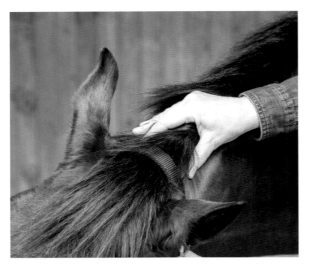

The horse's relaxation was profound, evidenced by his complete lowering of the head towards the ground, allowing me to access the tissues more effectively. However, you must exercise caution and avoid applying excessive depth that may irritate highly sensitive areas for the horse.

Fingertip Compression to Upper Cervical Area

Gently rotate the fingertips in a circular motion, moving around the upper cervical muscles located behind the head at the top of the neck. This is a tender area for most horses, so you might have to adjust the pressure a few times before you get it right. Alternatively, you might start by simply holding your hand steady over the area; this can be enough for the horse to know that you acknowledge its pain as we do in palpation also.

Fingertip Compression to Upper Cervical Area with Resting Head

This technique involves applying fingertip compression double-handed to the upper cervical muscles while the horse's head rests on your shoulder. It is more advanced owing to the horse's position, so act with caution.

Begin by gently positioning the horse's head on

your shoulder, considering your height and the size of the horse. Ensure the horse's head is not too elevated, as tilting the nose upwards excessively can cause the upper neck joints to close tightly.

Once the horse's head is comfortably resting on your shoulder, place the flat part of both hands over the targeted area to signal your presence. Then, gradually initiate a circular compression motion using your fingertips. This positioning of the horse's head allows the muscles to relax and soften while your shoulders bear the weight of its head. Only perform if comfortable to do so.

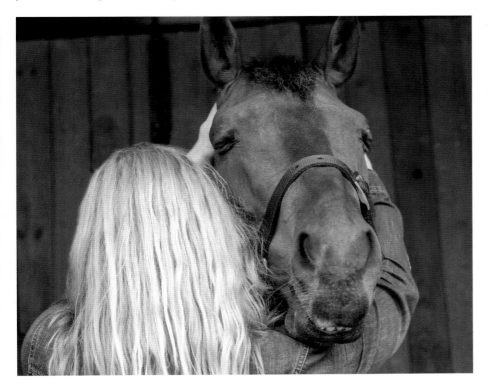

The horse's head resting on my shoulder, he is indicating complete relaxation with his eyes closed and a loose lip.

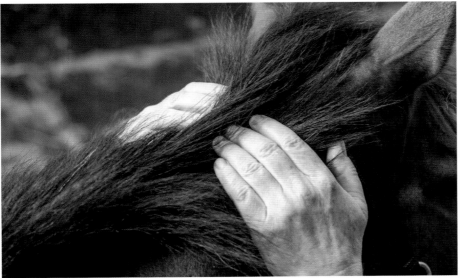

Letting the horse know my hands are resting on the area before starting the compressions with my fingertips.

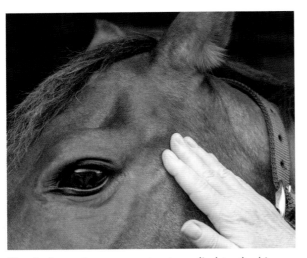

Gentle fingertip compression is applied to the hinge of the TMJ, but you can work all around the TMJ

Fingertip Compression to TMJ

Applying fingertip compressions to the temporomandibular joint (TMJ) area is highly effective in promoting relaxation and improving circulation in this often stagnant region. Continue performing the compressions for as long as the horse finds it comforting.

THE HORSE IN COMPLETE RELAXATION AFTER HEAD AND NECK WORK

This horse was so relaxed after receiving the compression work that I decided to gently place my hands on his forehead and see what happened. This is something for you to aim for with your own horse, indicating the immense benefit of your manual therapy work.

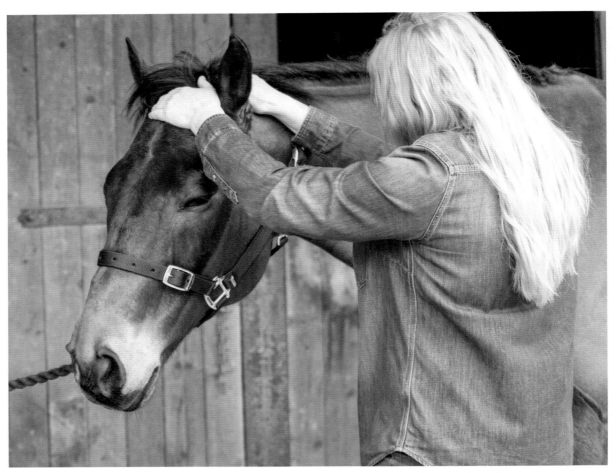

Gently placing my hands on the horse's forehead and upper cervical area, without pushing down, he began to close his eyes.

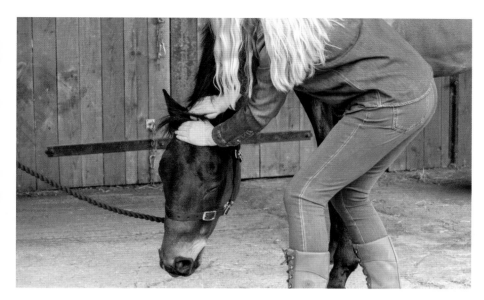

He continued to relax more deeply and lowered his head to the ground, and tightly closed his eyes. He stayed like this for a few minutes before raising his head and shaking it.

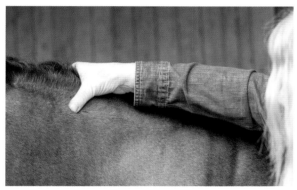

The hand position with the thumb on one side of the crest slowly compresses the tissue between the thumb, palm of the hand and fingers on the other side.

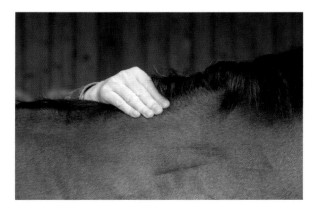

Showing the hand position with the fingers on the other side of the crest as the movement progresses upwards on the neck.

Compression to Body Areas – Single Handed

This is mostly performed on the horse's neck; it works well along the crest of the neck to relieve tension. Working up the neck from the withers to the poll, gently compress the tissue between thumb and fingers in a 'scooping' motion, similar to the palpation, but you focus on releasing some of the tension in the area rather than checking for its presence.

Single-handed compression with the flat knuckle to the muscle in the mid-section of the neck close to the shoulder edge (ventral serrate m.) helps with concussion the horse may receive, especially after working on firm ground; also, jumping horses hold a lot of tension here. You can also perform this to the upper portion of the neck on the crest (splenius m. and rhomboid m.) but avoid the cervical vertebrae itself.

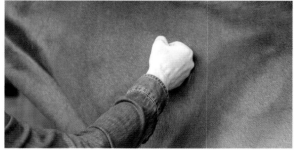

Applying single-handed compression to the neck muscle (ventral serrate m.).

Compression to Body Areas Double-Handed

Three areas on the horse lend themselves perfectly to double-handed compressions, performed in the same way as the single-handed, but it is a more intense technique. You will likely have to test your pressure on the lower edge of the shoulder (triceps m.) and hip flexor (tensor fascia lata m.) to suit the horse, as these areas are often tender due to absorbing concussion from the limbs. Repeat several times if necessary.

Many horses experience tension in the hamstring region and may lean into your hands, allowing for the opportunity to apply slightly firmer pressure by utilising your body weight for added force. However, if the horse pulls away or moves, it indicates that you are applying excessive depth and should make the necessary adjustments.

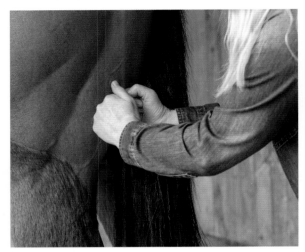

Apply the compression technique along the entire length of the hamstrings, commencing from the upper edge and progressing downwards towards the lower portion, as depicted in the image.

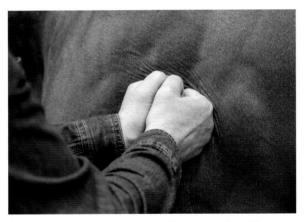

Applying the compression to the lower shoulder (triceps m.). Be careful with the technique so you do not nip the horse.

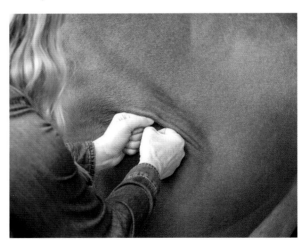

Applying the compression to the hip flexor (tensor fascia lata m.). This area can sometimes feel dry under your hand if there is insufficient circulation to the area.

FRICTION

What? The word 'friction' originates from the Latin word *fricare*, which means 'to rub'; it is a remedial technique used to increase circulation and release tight and stuck areas. The tissue is massaged to create friction and heat whilst stretching the fibres. It also helps to remove waste deposits and stimulate collagen fibres.

Where? It is very effective when performed over adhesions where the tissue feels like a rigid band under the skin. Adhesions are common along the horse's back. It is also useful over scar tissue to help with pliability, but the wound must have thoroughly healed first. Never perform over a place that is tender for the horse or to the horse's face. Only work on the area for a maximum of one minute to avoid bruising. The area should be warmed first by either compression or shaking techniques.

When? Only perform friction when the horse is not going to be ridden, because the nature of the technique means it will heat the tissue to the extent that it could cause inflammation as well as restore the tissue. This is fine if the horse is rested afterwards for at least 48 hours. Most beneficial within the sub-categories of: maintenance and remedial.

How? It is performed with the fingertips in small back-and-forth movements to penetrate the adhesion in the tissue. If the adhesion feels like a taut band of tissue, start at one end and perform the friction to the other end. If it feels like a knot, then apply to the centre of the knot and then around its edges.

Friction to an Adhesion on the Horse's Back

This is frequently needed in the back area due to saddle damage that has resulted in adhesions or scar tissue. This condition is often identified by white hairs, indicating the possibility of necrotic tissue or tissue death, although white hair is not always present.

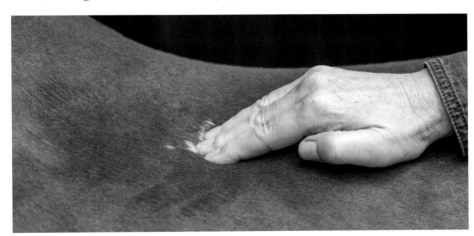

Once the adhesion is located – it is shown here under the white hair in the saddle region – the first movement is to push forward into the tissue and down with the fingertips.

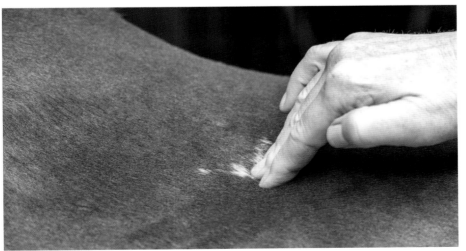

The second movement is to pull the tissue back, whereby the hand is raised slightly, and continue to repeat both movements to form the friction technique, along the length of adhesion.

Professional Case-Studies

This is an appropriate point in the book to say that my colleagues and I have observed remarkable transformations in horses through equine musculoskeletal (manual) therapy. I will highlight the profound effects it can have on horses by sharing information on three professional case studies from my records.

CASE STUDY ONE – JACK

Case Study Overview

This case study focuses on Jack, a six-year-old ex-racehorse who had been struggling with the challenges of being in racing, which was affecting his performance and overall quality of life. He was retired because he 'was not showing much promise on the track', but when he was rehomed, it was then that the new owner discovered he had possible sacroiliac injuries. Jack became a patient of my business partner, Therese Murphy, in her Equine Injury and Rehabilitation Clinic in Ireland.

Initial Assessment

At the outset of 2022, Jack exhibited muscular tension, restricted movement and muscle asymmetry in the pelvic region. When Jack was viewed from behind, the muscle asymmetry was evident and a sign that he was compensating for pain or weakness in his pelvis. Also, a lack of tone in the gluteal muscles was a sign that he could not engage the muscles of his hindquarter correctly. On dynamic assessment, he displayed the classic signs of 'bunny hopping', indicating sacroiliac pain. He also rested his hindquarters on the water drinker in the stable, and evidence of excrement on the walls both presented signs of sacroiliac pain. Regarding his emotional health, he had general unease due to the pain and irritability. Therese conducted a comprehensive assessment of Jack, carefully evaluating his history, the horse's posture, range of motion, dynamic assessment and response to palpation. She could then develop a customised plan for him targeting the specific areas of concern.

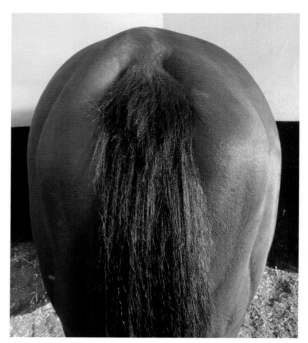

The image shows the extent of the asymmetry in Jack's musculature, including around the tuber sacrale, gluteal muscles and hamstring group. The left side displays considerably more pronounced muscling compared to the right. The twisted sacrum suggests a fall or injury. There is evidence of tail rubbing, as horses instinctively attempt to alleviate discomfort in the affected area.

Manual Therapy Intervention

Drawing upon a range of remedial therapy techniques, supported by equine kinesiology taping and electrotherapy, Therese focused on promoting relaxation and pain relief, releasing the tension in the overdeveloped muscles, and improving circulation. Careful attention was given to addressing the hindquarter areas likely to have experienced an injury.

Progress and Transformation

Over the course of several treatments and gentle in-hand exercises, along with daily turn-out, a remarkable transformation took place. Jack gradually started exhibiting enhanced flexibility, increased range of motion and improved overall muscle tone. The horse's demeanour notably shifted from restlessness and unease to a more relaxed, contented state.

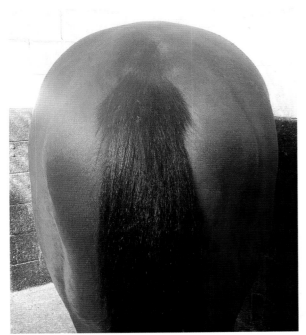

This image clearly demonstrates noticeable improvements in his musculature, with increased symmetry and a straighter sacrum.

Outcome

Jack's performance and overall health were greatly improved, and he is now able to enjoy riding club activities with his owner and regular maintenance massages from her. This illuminating case study is evident that equine manual therapy can be a catalyst for transformative change in horses with the right approach and expert care.

CASE STUDY TWO – ESME

Case Study Overview

This case study focuses on Esme, a fourteen-year-old skewbald mare. In 2018 Millicent Sword first met Esme, at which time there was no deviation to her nose, it occurred a year later in 2019. The veterinarian thought it was possibly an allergy, but the owner decided that Esme was the perfect candidate for manual therapy with Millicent (Millie), who is an experienced manual therapist and also works in my training company as an administrator, assessor and researcher.

Initial Assessment

In 2019 a thorough assessment revealed that Esme had sensitivity in her sinus area and a great deal of tension in her nostrils and also her hyoid apparatus (a collection of bones and cartilage located in the neck that supports and anchors the tongue, larynx and other structures involved in swallowing and vocalisation). She had limited facial movement and a raised left-side frontal bone compared to the right, with muscle tension to the left also. Muscle tension was also found in her neck and hindquarter muscles.

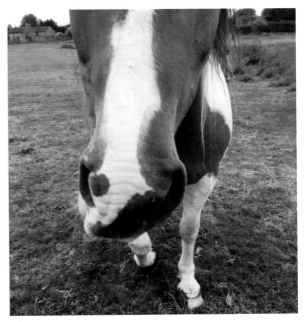

Evidence of the muzzle deviation.

Manual Therapy Intervention

Esme had two treatments with Millie in September 2019 and another in November, whereby the deviation in her nose and the overall tension was much improved and barely noticeable, just a little deviation.

Progress and Transformation

Esme continued to progress and receives regular manual therapy from Millie and, on her visit in May 2020, she noticed that Esme had some fibrous tissue (a form of scar tissue) across her nose and muzzle but the deviation was much improved as was the sensitivity.

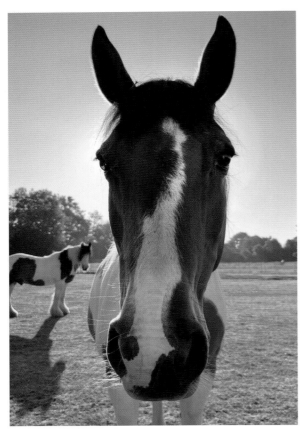

A significant improvement in the symmetry.

Outcome

Esme enjoys her ridden activities and continues to receive six-monthly manual therapy treatments from Millie to keep her musculature supple and free from tension. The right expert support made Esme a happier and more comfortable mare.

CASE STUDY THREE – PUDDLE

Case Study Overview

This case study focuses on Puddle, a twelve-year-old thoroughbred ex-racehorse. He was trained and raced until he was around four and ran six races. No explanation was given as to why he retired from racing. His current owner purchased Puddle after he finished racing and has done very little with him apart from the occasional hack, and he has not been ridden in the last two and a half years. Around two years ago, he received hock injections. He became a project for Marie Stephenson, owing to being in the same yard. Marie is an experienced manual therapist and also works in my training company as an assessor, student liaison and instructor.

Initial Assessment

After conducting a comprehensive assessment of Puddle in 2023, Marie discovered pronounced muscle asymmetry, muscle atrophy and regions of muscular tension. Puddle also exhibited sacroiliac issues. During palpation, Marie observed persistent pain in the hocks, despite previous injections, evident from Puddle's stance and the presence of heat in the area.

Manual Therapy Intervention

Over a period of a couple of months, Marie provided Puddle with manual therapy treatments focusing on the shoulders, back and hindquarters to help with asymmetry and the deviation in the spine. Also, some electrotherapy work on the hocks. The owner

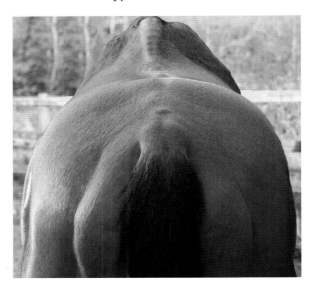

The image clearly shows asymmetry in Puddle's musculature – the right wither is significantly larger than the left. The spine deviates to the right. From the image, vertebral column damage would be a consideration.

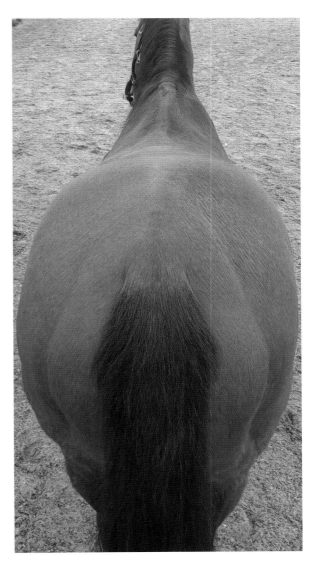

This image is taken after the manual therapy intervention, although at a slightly different angle, it shows the spine is straightening due to the muscle tension being removed. The wither asymmetry is also progressing.

also gives the horse regular therapy. Marie also gave the owner some gentle in-hand exercises to perform.

Progress and Transformation

The progress has been very beneficial, and Puddle's muscles are starting to show signs of becoming more balanced, the spine is straighter, and the shoulder and wither asymmetry is an ongoing process.

Outcome

Puddle's owner takes him for in-hand walks. He has a changed diet and a new bit following a bit and bridle consultation. The saddle has also been checked in readiness for when he will be ridden again. Puddle is a much-loved horse with no rush from the owner to begin work. A difference can already be seen in his muscular stature with a combination of manual therapy, diet change, tack assessment and commitment from the owner.

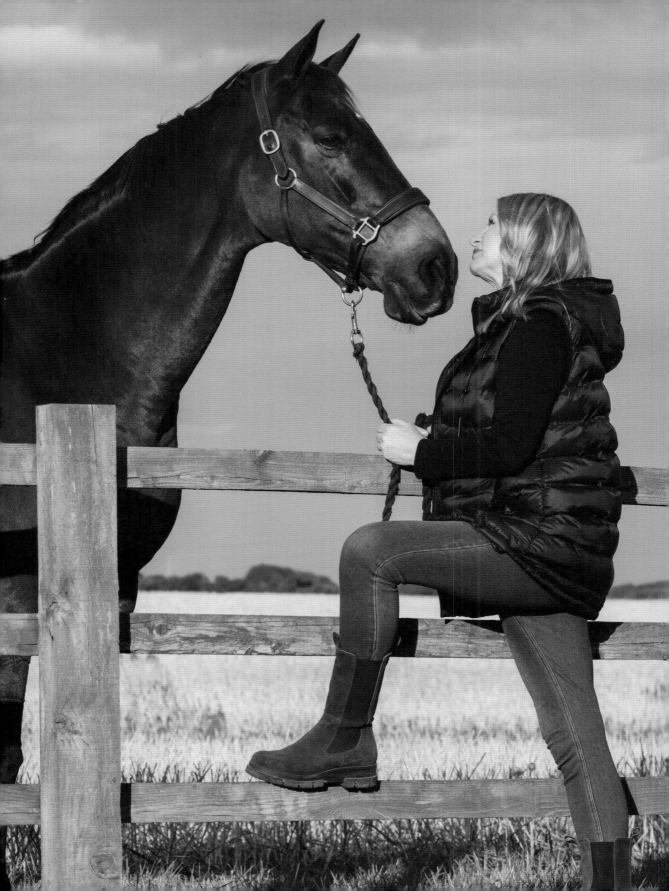

CHAPTER 8

Correct Supportive Exercise

Expanding on the information provided in Chapter 4, this chapter highlights that by engaging in correct supportive exercise designed to strengthen horses' muscles, improve their balance, coordination, and flexibility, you can help your horse avoid injury and perform at their best. Moreover, incorporating appropriate exercises within a comprehensive training regimen adopts a strategic approach and well-structured framework with the aim of minimising the risk of injuries and setbacks in performance.

Before delving into specific corrective exercise, it is crucial to address certain key factors that form the foundation of your training. These considerations should not be overlooked and include:

The Training Surface and Time of Day

The best surfaces for horse training depend on exercise and individual needs. They should provide some give for muscle development and slightly firmer surfaces for bone strength. Avoid extremes like deep sand or concrete. Grass is natural, forgiving, and offers good traction while being easy on the horse's joints, unless very firm in summer months. It is ideal for light work, lunging and horses recovering from injury. Sand and rubber surfaces offer traction and bounce, making them suitable for dressage and jumping. Combining different surfaces can improve strength, balance and fitness. Regularly check and maintain surfaces for safety. Water exercise, like hydrotherapy, can be beneficial with proper training and precautions. Training during the day when horses are alert is recommended, considering temperature extremes. Observe your horse's behaviour and adjust the training schedule accordingly. Quiet environments help maintain focus and significantly impact training outcomes.

The Equipment

TRAINING AIDS

In the world of horse training, various aids are available to assist trainers in their pursuit of improving a horse's performance. However, it is essential to approach the use of training aids with caution, as their improper use can harm and hinder the horse's wellbeing, which I have much evidence of seeing in the industry. While I personally prefer simpler aids like a lunge line or long rein for certain exercises or some tactile stimulation of the hindquarters with a simple tail bandage safely fitted to a roller or girth, it is important to acknowledge that training aids should never be seen as a substitute for proper training techniques, consistent groundwork and a strong foundation of communication and trust between the horse and the trainer.

If you do choose to incorporate training aids into your training regimen, it is crucial to do so under the guidance of knowledgeable instruction. Seek the assistance of a qualified trainer who can provide proper guidance on their application and usage. Never fit them to the horse or its tack with guesswork, otherwise considerable harm can be caused to the horse that may not be undone.

It is also recommended to closely monitor the horse's movements and responses when using a training aid to ensure that it is not causing undue restriction or discomfort. Each horse is unique, and it is crucial to be attentive to their individual needs and wellbeing throughout the training process.

By taking a balanced approach and using training aids responsibly, you can potentially leverage any benefits while safeguarding the welfare and wellbeing of your horse.

Poles

Pole work is beneficial for horses as it helps to improve their balance, coordination and athleticism. Using poles on the ground can assist with proprioception, which is the horse's self-awareness of where its limbs are; this sense develops over time, and pole work is excellent for young horses that are developing this sense or those that have had injuries to their limbs. Balance and coordination benefit from pole work, and core and back strength can benefit. Additionally, pole work can be used as a fun and varied way to exercise a horse, which can help to keep them mentally stimulated.

Cavaletti is a type of exercise for horses that involves walking, trotting or cantering over slightly raised poles, in hand or ridden, which I regularly use in my programmes. These poles are typically set at a lower height than regular jumps and are arranged in a line or in a pattern designed to help improve a horse's balance, coordination and jumping technique. It can also be used to develop a horse's strength and flexibility and to improve its ability to use its hindquarters effectively. Walking over cavaletti helps to stimulate joint fluid; it is, there-fore, useful for a horse with arthritic joints as long as it is not overdone, which would exacerbate the horse's pain and discomfort. Cavaletti improves the horse's overall fitness and can be used as a warm-up or cool-down exercise before and after riding.

Your Specialist Skills Requirements

As well as being proficient in riding, lunging is considered a specialist skill because it requires a combination of knowledge, technique and experience to do it correctly.

A person lunging a horse needs to have a good understanding of how to communicate with the horse, how to use the lunge line and whip effectively, and how to read the horse's body language and adjust their commands accordingly. Additionally, lunging a horse requires a good understanding of the different gaits and how to ask for them correctly. The person lunging a horse should be able to differentiate between the horse's natural gait and when the horse is running away or pushing too hard.

Very often, I see people lunging horses whilst looking at their mobile phones; this means their eyes are down, which is a command in lunging for the horse to slow down, but when they use a whip at the same time, asking the horse to move forward, this is very confusing for the horse and incorrect.

A simple lunge line fitted to a cavesson noseband or a lunging roller is sufficient, as it encourages the horse to use its body naturally without learning to lean and move against resistance. If you need to lunge off a bridle for added control, it is best not to fit it directly onto the bit because this tilts the jaw and is not suitable for the horse; instead, use a lunging attachment for the bridle.

The best way to lunge a horse is to do so freely; the horse will learn to support itself in self-carriage, maintain good shape and be balanced. Lunging can only be done correctly with proper training and experience.

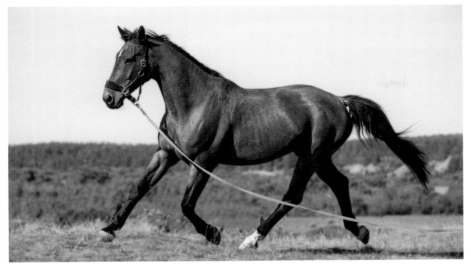

Lunging a horse freely is advantageous to enable the horse to find a balanced, natural movement so muscles can develop correctly without tension. In addition, the horse's face does not show any sign of pain. This is very positive.

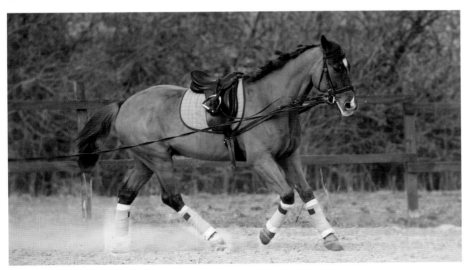

The training aids force the horse into a restricted, tense frame. The horse's face shows signs of pain with foam at the mouth. This lunging can cause muscle damage and is not favourable.

The horse pictured right is demonstrating being lunged freely using simple equipment. It is tracking up, bending correctly on the circle, engaging its hindquarters and working uphill. The horse is holding a good posture, and the forelimb and shoulder are free and not restricted, allowing a good range of motion.

The horse pictured above is restricted in its neck and locked into position with training aids. The forelimb range of motion is limited because the horse is on the forehand with a high-head carriage. The hindquarters are engaging, but there is tension in the front end due to the restrictive training aids. The core is weak because its movement is not natural. It is unbalanced

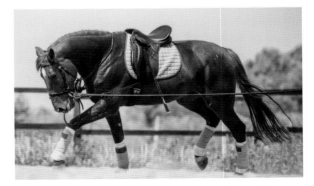

The core and back are not used correctly, as the horse's frame is tight and tied in with side reins. The horse's face is showing signs of pain. This can cause muscle damage and is not favourable.

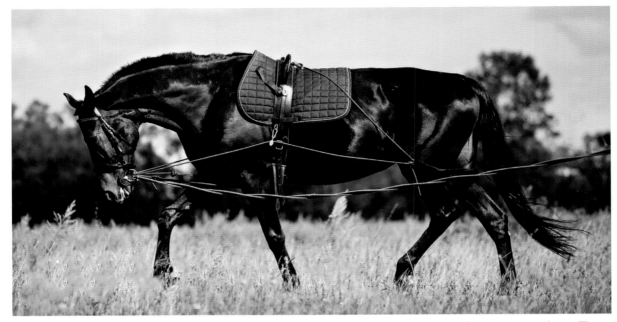

The back is hollow and weak and under strain. The core is weak. The horse's face is showing signs of pain. This can cause muscle damage and is not favourable.

and not bending correctly on the circle.

The same horse on the previous page, is overbending being lunged; its neck is extremely overbent with a high level of tension in its poll and neck muscles. There is too much pressure. The hindquarters are not used effectively as the neck is restricted, so the horse cannot move forward with power and impulsion. The hindlimbs have a limited range of motion, not coming under the horse or tracking up.

The horse pictured above is locked into a frame; the training aid pulley system is restricting its entire structure; it is overbending due to the tension in the training aid restricting the forelimb range of motion, resulting in neck tension that can be seen as it moves on the forehand. Due to being locked in, the horse cannot use its hindquarters correctly. The hindquarters are very weak, and the hindlimbs are not pushing the horse forward and coming underneath it.

CHECKS FOR HORSE AND RIDER

The Horse

Before embarking on a new training programme, it is advantageous to have a musculoskeletal therapist give the horse a complete check-over beforehand to ensure the horse has the best chance to succeed. This might include checking for pre-existing conditions or injuries that may affect the training to ensure they have healed correctly. Also, ensure that your horse's feet, teeth and tack are the best they can be before you start the training programme.

Create a health record for the horse, recording the baseline figures of the vital signs, which are temperature, heart rate and respiration. Take these weekly to help identify if they are consistent or fluctuate, which will identify any potential health issues early on that might impede the training. Vital signs will also tell you how your horse is responding to the training. Learn how to do this correctly.

Take photographs or video footage of your horse before you start; this is your baseline, and plan to take more at specific intervals – usually, four weeks

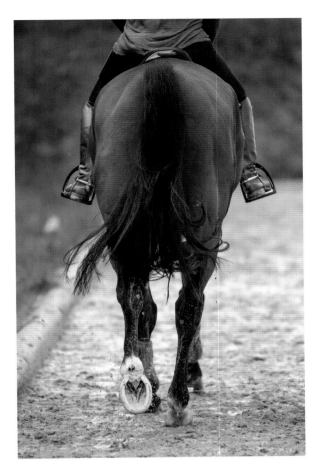

This rider and horse both need manual therapy to correct imbalances. If left unchecked, both will develop compensatory patterns in their bodies that will be difficult to fix the longer they continue.

apart – which will be your benchmark and identify any improvements or failings. This should comprise how it looks, in particular its muscle balance; you can use the flex curve to take impressions. Also, video the horse in movement, without a rider and with a rider to assess it dynamically.

Ensure the horse's diet is suitable. Often, they are overfed for their needs – mainly too much concentrated grain feed. Good quality forage is the best starting point, which can be built on if necessary.

The Rider

When riding a horse, the rider needs to be well-balanced, because an off-balance rider can disrupt the horse's balance and cause it to become unsteady or unresponsive. Additionally, an off-balance rider may have difficulty communicating their commands effectively to the horse, leading to confusion or misunderstandings. Furthermore, a balanced rider is likelier to stay seated when the horse makes sudden movements. This can prevent accidents and injuries to both the rider and the horse.

Assess yourself to determine if you have aches, pains or body asymmetries when riding. Ask a friend to film you whilst riding, as this will show any asymmetries. You can then get the required help. It is preferable to avoid riding if you are in pain and cannot sit correctly as the horse will compensate; you can do in-hand exercising instead or this is a good opportunity to perform your manual therapy.

This asymmetrical rider above would place more weight through her left hip, femur and lower leg, weighing the horse more on its left and a stronger contact on the left. The rider's right leg is placed further forward, giving inconsistent aids. The saddle will be unstable and move on the horse's back. The rider's back is hollow, indicating her pelvis is tilting forward, which places more weight on the front of the saddle. This is not a desirable ridden image, but it is common and often far worse asymmetries are seen.

The Correct Supportive Exercise Programme

We assume that all the relevant checks have been made with both the horse and rider to ensure you are both ready to start the programme. By taking these measures, you have created the best possible foundation for your success and to reach your full potential, which needs clear goals, patience, consistency and not taking the horse beyond its capabilities. Your role is to create a well-structured plan with the individual goals, exercises, rest periods and the stages when you will monitor progress.

However, firstly, you must accurately assess your horse's current level of fitness and ability without it being forced to do anything. What comes naturally for the horse is always a good starting point, and it does with enjoyment rather than something it finds difficult and overtires. Always be mindful of any previous or ongoing injuries or conditions that might need injury prevention training, which means you avoid training that places any stress on the injury or condition. The horse must be exercised correctly in any programme with enough rest and recovery.

The following are examples of your correct supportive exercise programme goals. Your horse will certainly fall into one or more of these:

- Pre-training
- Strength and conditioning training
- Continuation training
- Rehabilitation training
- Recurring injury prevention
- To improve the horse 'on the bit'
- To improve collection and balance
- To improve lunging work
- To improve in-hand work
- To improve the communication between you and the horse
- To strengthen the horse's core and back
- To improve lateral work
- To improve dressage or jumping techniques
- To incorporate more warm-up and cool-down
- To improve in-hand work.

Once you have established your goals, it is important to write them down, fully commit to them, and create a plan for the exercises you need to do, along with how often. This will allow you to develop a supportive and effective exercise programme tailored to your specific goals and horse's needs. By following this approach, you can increase your chances of success and achieve meaningful progress towards your desired outcomes.

DIFFICULTY VERSUS INTENSITY

Difficulty and intensity are related concepts but have distinct meanings in different contexts.

Difficulty in horse exercises refers to the level of complexity or challenge involved in performing a particular exercise or task not only by the horse but the rider too. It encompasses the mental and physical demands to execute the movement correctly. Factors that contribute to the difficulty of an exercise for a horse may include coordination, balance, collection, lateral movements, transitions or jumping technicalities. A difficult exercise for a horse might require precise timing, coordination of multiple body parts or advanced training to achieve proper execution.

Intensity refers to the level of physical exertion or effort required by the horse and rider to perform the exercise. It focuses on the degree of physical demand placed on the horse's body during the execution of the movement. Intensity can be influenced by factors such as speed, duration, resistance or height in exercises such as galloping, extended trotting, collected canter, jumping over high obstacles or engaging in fast-paced activities such as eventing or racing. High-intensity exercises often require significant cardiovascular and muscular effort from the horse and not all horses achieve this level other than those working professionally.

THE INTENSITY PHASES OF EXERCISE

Any training programme is gradual to help minimise injury and to enable the horse's body to adjust to the changes in exercise types and levels. There are no shortcuts: sudden changes and increases in work can result in muscle injuries, time off and a return to the beginning.

For example, when building fitness (conditioning) in the programme, duration and intensity should never be increased together. One at a time, allowing for a two- to three-week adaptation before increasing the other. So, if gallop is introduced into the programme, gallop at the same duration and intensity for two to three weeks before galloping uphill, which is more strenuous and, as such, increases in intensity.

Always monitor the horse's progress and adjust the programme accordingly to ensure it is not overworked or at risk of injury. Ensure it is ready to progress to the next phase, otherwise good work done in a phase might be undone if you progress too soon.

Pre-training – the horse will likely be in the initial phase to low-intensity phase.
Strength and conditioning – the horse is likely to be in the low-intensity phase to medium-intensity phase.
Continuation – the horse is likely to be in the medium-intensity phase but, with certain professions, it might include some high-intensity phase work.
Rehabilitation – this is a specific exercise to restore the horse to its former condition through very specific therapy with strength and conditioning work, usually starting at the low-intensity or the initial phase depending on the severity of the injury.

Initial Phase

This phase typically involves basic exercises that help the horse's confidence, become familiar with being ridden, which may be different to what it has been used to, improve its balance, and be a foundation on which to build its fitness level gradually. Incorporating:

Walking – lots of walking helps to improve the horse's balance, especially if done so in straight lines, large circles, through cones, or over cavaletti.
Lunging or long lining – again, this helps with balance, fitness and when worked at a controlled pace, allows you to see how your horse moves.

In-hand work – this helps improve the horse's flexibility and coordination and builds trust between the horse and handler.
Education – depending on the age of the horse or if training from one profession to another, such as racehorse to riding horse, some basic education skills may have been missing or done differently. Such as learning to mount from a block, equipment and tack it might not be familiar with, desensitising such as working in an arena, getting used to farm equipment, voice commands, basic manoeuvring on the ground.

Low-Intensity Phase

Low-intensity work for a horse typically involves exercises that require minimal exertion and stress on the horse's body. This type of work is often used for warm-up, cool-down or recovery periods between higher-intensity workouts. This phase also starts fitness and strength building whilst minimising the risk of injury or fatigue. Incorporating:

Walking – this can be used for warm-up and cool-down periods. It is also a good form of exercise for horses that are recovering from injuries or are returning to work after time off.
Trotting – is a slightly more intense exercise than walking, but still considered a low-intensity workout. It can help improve a horse's cardiovascular fitness and muscle tone without placing too much strain on the body.
Lunging – doing this in walk, trot and progressing to canter will help balance, coordination, flexibility and fitness.
Hill work – walking or trotting up and down hills for a short period can be a low-intensity way to build strength and endurance without putting too much strain on the horse's body.
Pole work – exercises involving ground poles can help improve a horse's balance, coordination and footwork. They can be set up in a variety of patterns and at varying heights to create a low-intensity workout for the horse.

Medium-Intensity Phase

This typically involves exercises that require moderate exertion and can help improve the horse's cardiovascular fitness (condition), strength and endurance. These types of workouts are often used to help a horse progress in its strength and conditioning training and prepare for higher-intensity work if this is required. However, many horses will only ever remain in the medium-intensity phase and not reach the high-intensity phase unless they are working horses in an equestrian profession or have heavy competition schedules. Incorporating:

Trotting and cantering – these are exercises that can help improve a horse's fitness level and build muscle strength. These gaits can be used for longer periods of time than in low-intensity work and can be done on various surfaces, such as flat ground or hills.

Interval training – this involves alternating between periods of intensity in exercise and rest which could be mostly in medium-intensity with short bursts of high-intensity then rest. This type of training can help improve a horse's stamina and endurance and can be done through various exercises such as trotting or cantering with intermittent changes in gait or incorporating some pole work or a gymnastic course.

Hill work – this can be a medium-intensity workout for a horse, especially when done at a faster pace or with steeper inclines. This exercise can help improve the horse's cardiovascular fitness, strength and balance.

Jumping – this can help improve a horse's coordination, balance and overall fitness level. It can be done with low-height jumps and gradually increased as the horse progresses in its training, but the horse should not be jumping at higher heights constantly – even if it can do so – because this can be very damaging on joints.

Dressage training – this involves precise movements and exercises that can help improve a horse's balance, suppleness and responsiveness to the rider's aids. This type of training can be considered medium-intensity, as it requires focused attention and can be physically demanding, so you must ensure warm-up and cool-down as well as lots of rest in between exercises.

High-Intensity Phase

This phase is done sparingly and carefully, and you must check for any injury or if the horse struggles with this phase check its fitness and skills. Typically, it involves exercises that require significant exertion. This type of workout is often used to improve the horse's performance in competition or to prepare for intense physical activities, such as eventing, racing or endurance riding. You must check for any injuries during this phase and monitor how the horse is coping with the level of intensity. You must also ensure plenty of rest periods. Incorporating:

Galloping – this involves the horse running at a fast pace. It can be done on a track, in a field and can help improve a horse's cardiovascular fitness and speed.

Interval training – this is when the periods of high-intensity exercise are longer and more intense than in medium-intensity workouts. For example, interval training can involve short bursts of galloping or cantering followed by rest periods.

Jumping course/gymnastic course – this involves a series of poles and jumps of varying heights. This type of workout can help improve a horse's jumping technique, speed and agility.

Dressage – increasing the exercise demand for the horse or duration than in the medium-intensity phase.

Long hack – a long hack with varying terrain, hill work, obstacles, areas for gallop, etc., can be varied high-intensity exercise for a horse.

Endurance riding – involving the horse covering long distances over varying terrain. This type of workout requires a high level of cardiovascular fitness and stamina. The horse needs to be well prepared for this.

The Correct Supportive Exercise

Now that you are prepared, it is time to commence a programme of correct supportive exercise that can be performed in conjunction with manual therapy and other essential management components discussed in this book, necessary for properly training your horse.

IN-HAND WORK

In-hand work is often overlooked and, through scientific studies, we know that controlled flat work (unridden, progressing to ridden work) is extremely beneficial for the horse in several ways. It can develop balance and co-ordination, strengthen muscles, and it also helps to build trust and develop a stronger bond when the person and horse work together on the ground. I have seen many horses benefit from a mental break from schooling work when working in-hand, making them more enthusiastic about their ridden work.

Every exercise performed in hand must be con-trolled exercise and not rushed.

The horse should be led on a long rein, because you want its head in a naturally lower position. The horse needs to work out what it is doing when approaching the poles and move through them at its own pace lifting its feet at the same time.

In-hand work is beneficial during any exercise programme and any intensity; it is an excellent groundwork exercise and often not done enough.

Walking Over a Series of Ground Poles

This is a popular exercise whereby the horse must be walking comfortably over a single pole first and then a series of poles. The pole distance apart must be correct depending on the size and stride length of the horse – usually between seventy centimetres and one metre apart. The method of placing the pole three-person steps apart is not accurate. You should know the exact measurement in person steps or using a measuring device as correct for your horse.

The benefits are:

- Improves balance and coordination by encour-aging the horse to lift its legs higher and place them more deliberately, which can also improve its proprioception.
- Enhances flexibility and range of motion because it requires the horse to stretch its muscles and

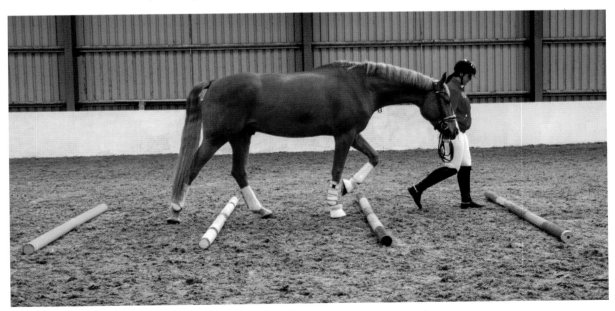

Six ground poles are placed evenly apart according to the horse's stride length.

joints, thus helping to increase flexibility and range of motion.

- Develops strength by helping to strengthen a horse's muscles, particularly those in their legs and core, as they work to maintain their balance and stride.
- Engages the mind because it is mentally stimulating for them as they must pay attention to where they are placing their feet and adjust their stride accordingly. This can help to keep them focused and engaged during training sessions. Also, they are more responsive to the handler's cues.

Walking over a Series of Raised Poles

Walking over raised poles (cavaletti) can provide additional benefits to a horse's physical and mental well-being compared to walking over flat poles. Here are some reasons why:

- Enhances muscle development by walking over raised cavaletti poles – it requires the horse to lift their legs higher, flex their joints more, and use their muscles differently than when walking over ground poles. This can help build strength and develop specific muscle groups, especially in the hindquarters, shoulders and back.
- Improves coordination and balance, because the raised cavaletti poles require the horse to pay closer attention to their foot placement and adjust their stride accordingly. This can also improve their overall proprioception.
- Increases joint flexibility – the higher clearance over the poles encourages the horse to flex and extend its joints more, which can improve joint mobility and flexibility.
- Builds confidence by successfully navigating the raised cavaletti poles, which can be a confidence-building experience for horses. As they become more comfortable with the exercise, they may start to feel more confident in their abilities, which can translate to other areas of their training.

As the horse progresses, gradually increase the height of the poles. If performing this exercise while riding, ensure the horse has a long rein and plenty of freedom for its head, similar to when being led. Avoid interfering with the horse and allow it to walk over the poles without encouragement.

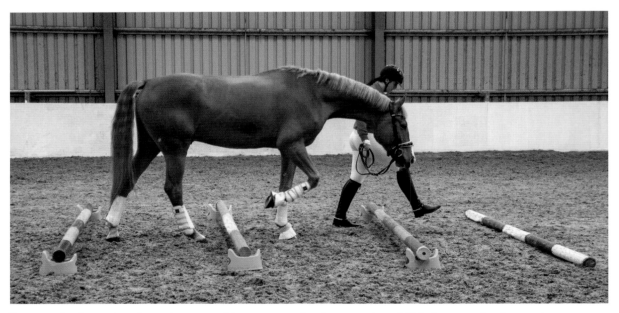

Four cavaletti are placed evenly apart, with two ground poles at each end. This is strengthening work performed with the poles from fetlock to mid-cannon bone height but never above knee height.

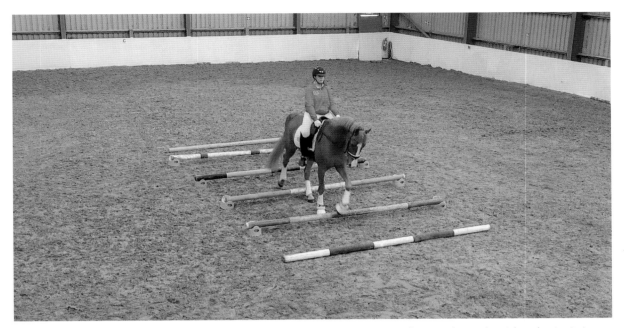

Demonstrating riding in a walk over a series of cavaletti. There is no interference from the rider, she is sitting straight and looking ahead.

Walking Uphill and Downhill

This serves as a strengthening and conditioning exercise for horses. It is important to note that horses should not be exercised on steep inclines unless it is part of a rehabilitation programme under clinical supervision. However, walking up and down a hill with a steady incline of around twenty metres in length, for a duration of ten to twenty minutes, can be considered a low- to high-intensity exercise depending on the horse's fitness level. Initially, these exercises are performed in-hand, and a horse should only be ridden uphill and downhill once it can comfortably perform the exercise in-hand without the additional strain of carrying a rider.

Walking Uphill: This exercise encourages the horse to shift its body weight towards the hindquarters, lightening the forehand. It is particularly effective for strengthening the hindquarters, including the lumbosacral junction. Additionally, it helps develop shoulder and limb strength, although its primary focus is on the hindquarters.

Walking uphill offers several benefits for the horse:

- Builds strength and endurance – walking uphill requires the horse to work harder against gravity, thereby building muscle strength and cardiovascular endurance.
- Promotes weight loss – walking uphill can burn more calories compared to walking on flat ground, which can be beneficial for horses that need to lose weight or maintain a healthy weight. However, if the horse is not at its required weight, hill work should be limited.

To increase the intensity of the exercise, poles can be added. Placing two or three poles at two strides apart requires the horse to pay closer attention to its foot placement, enhancing balance, coordination, joint flexibility and mobility.

Walking Downhill: This part of the exercise focuses on balance and coordination, as it challenges the horse to resist gravity during downhill locomotion. It stimulates the activation of the abdominal muscles and strengthens the core stabilisers which, in turn, assists the neck and back muscles.

It is important to note that walking downhill can

place a significant amount of strain on a horse's legs and joints, particularly if they are unfamiliar with the terrain or have pre-existing injuries or conditions. Therefore, it is crucial to introduce this exercise gradually and closely monitor the horse's behaviour and gait to ensure their comfort and the absence of pain. Furthermore, walking downhill should only be done under the supervision of an experienced handler.

Here are a few more benefits of walking downhill:

Improves coordination – walking downhill requires the horse to effectively use its hindquarters to control its stride and slow its descent. This can enhance its coordination and balance, making it more agile and responsive when ridden.

Develops bone density – the impact of the horse's feet hitting the ground while walking downhill stimulates the growth of bone tissue, improving bone density and strength.

Exercise for Re-setting the Horse's Balance

A horse's balance system can be improved through specific exercises that focus on improving its proprioception, because this is crucial for a horse's balance, coordination and overall movement. Young horses often have poor proprioception until it develops, and they are given exercises to support it and with more experienced horses, their balance system can become overloaded and require support to reset it.

Standing Square Over a Pole: A beneficial static exercise for horses encourages them to stand on either side of a pole. This exercise focuses on improving proprioception and balance, aiding in resetting the

Notice how the horse is standing with its body swayed towards the right. Its hind limbs are also further apart. Once the horse is settled in this position, it should be left there for as long as necessary. Eventually, with practice, it should stand more balanced.

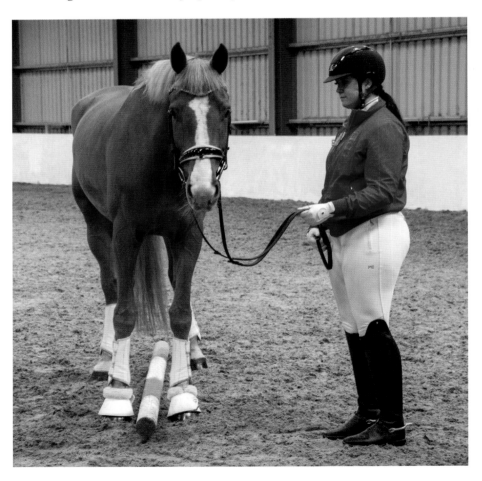

horse's balance system at any stage of training or age. Additionally, it provides relaxation for the horse and stimulates the parasympathetic nervous system, similar to the effects of manual therapy. I first encountered this totally by accident when a horse I was working with adopted this stance in the field by placing its legs on either side of a large branch, I watched it from afar and was astounded at the results, the horse looked as if it was falling asleep. This was a horse that was finding it very difficult to cope with the training and competition demands of the owner.

You might notice that the horse cannot stand squarely – and that is fine as, eventually, by practising the exercise, the horse should stand more squarely when performing it. Do not force the horse into a square position, as how it stands is part of the balance system, and if the horse finds it difficult to stand over the pole, ask a helper to gently and slowly slide the pole between the horse's legs from the front but with caution as you do not want to frighten or knock the horse when doing this, as it will not be compliant in the future and the helper is in a vulnerable position.

Other exercises that can help with the balance of the horse include:

- Pole work, ground poles or cavaletti style.
- Hill work can help balance, as the horse works to distribute its weight evenly across all four limbs.
- Lateral work, such as leg-yielding or shoulder-in, can help improve a horse's balance and coordination. These exercises require the horse to shift its weight from one side to the other, which can help improve its proprioception and overall balance too.
- Gymnastic exercises involving jumping or gymnastics, such as gridwork or bounce exercises, can help improve a horse's balance and coordination by forcing it to adjust its stride length and foot placement to navigate the obstacles.

RIDDEN WORK

Once the horse is established with in-hand pole work, it can progress to ridden work with poles.

But returning to in-hand work as part of a horse's training programme is beneficial; it gives the horse the opportunity to move its body in a balanced way but without carrying the weight of a rider. This is very beneficial for its wellbeing.

Sequences of Ground Poles

There are many variations of ground pole work – some very similar to others, and some can be rather confusing. I keep mine as simple as possible, ensuring the horse has enough to focus on and uses most of its body without over-phasing it. This exercise is more aimed at strength, conditioning and continuation training. Depending on how complex the sequences are and how close the poles are placed together, makes angles more acute and, therefore, more difficult for the horse. How long the horse is exercised over them denotes the intensity.

As such, I cannot give definitive guidelines on the difficulty and intensity, as I do not know your horse, but it depends on the level of skill and fitness of the horse and you. At all times, you must monitor how you and the horse are coping and adjust where necessary.

Working through any sequence of ground pole exercises is specifically beneficial for:

- Improving coordination, because the sequences of poles require the horse to navigate between and around obstacles, which can help to improve their coordination, balance and proprioception. This can translate to better performance in other areas, such as jumping or dressage.
- Strengthening muscles due to the action of lifting and manoeuvring their legs over poles and around obstacles can help to strengthen the muscles in the horse's legs, back, hindquarters and neck. This can improve their overall strength and athleticism.
- Encouraging consistent stride length, because pole work obstacles are typically spaced a consistent distance apart. This encourages the horse to maintain a consistent stride length and rhythm, which can help develop a more balanced and efficient gait. This can make it easier for the horse to

maintain a steady pace and rhythm in other exercises or disciplines, such as jumping or dressage.

- Encouraging engagement and impulsion, because the horse is required to engage its hindquarters and move with more impulsion and maintain a rhythm over the poles, it engages its core muscles and hindquarters, which can help improve overall strength and power.
- Increases focus, because horses can become bored and distracted if they are doing the same exercise repeatedly. Working over and around sequences of poles provides variety and stimulates the horse's mind, which can increase their focus, engagement and enjoyment in their work.

The following exercises use ground poles for all categories of training – pre-training, strength and conditioning, continuation and rehabilitation – depending on how they are performed. Always incorporate the warm-up and cool-down with some walking, trotting, cantering (depending on the stage for the horse), and two or three of the following exercises to add variety and stimulation to the strength and conditioning training, but to not tire the horse.

It is important to note that bending around poles requires training and practice to develop the necessary skills and coordination for both the horse and rider. Safety measures should be taken to ensure the horse's wellbeing, such as using lightweight poles that can easily fall if touched and providing adequate space for manoeuvring between the poles.

The Labyrinth: This exercise requires six poles placed on the ground so the horse can walk over them diagonally, around the outside and also inside the poles in a serpentine shape. The closer together the poles are placed, the more difficult the exercise is due to acute turns.

This is very beneficial for all-around strengthening of the deeper postural muscles and the superficial movement muscles.

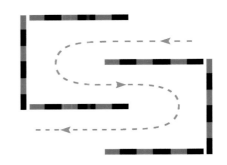

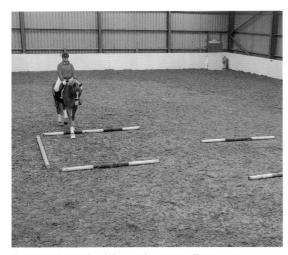

Approaching the labyrinth in a walk.

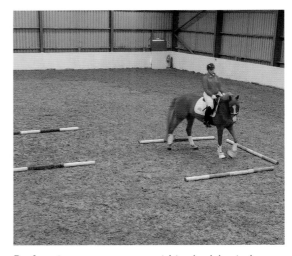

Performing an acute turn within the labyrinth.

The Serpentine: This exercise requires three or more poles placed on the centre line. Placed closer together requires a tighter serpentine, therefore, is more difficult, whilst a greater distance between the poles is less difficult, as you will perform the serpentine deeper.

This is very beneficial for the pelvic muscles, the back and abdominals and the thoracic sling in the front end of the horse.

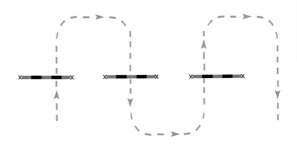

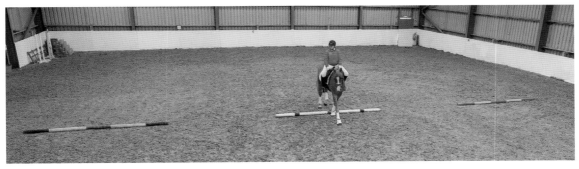

Walking over the centre pole of the serpentine.

The Serpentine Twist: This exercise requires four poles spaced in a square shape with an angled pole. The intensity depends on whether the exercise progresses from walk to trot, and the difficulty depends on if you ride a deep-twisting serpentine or an acute twist. You can perform half-halts also in front of poles to increase the difficulty and intensity. Some poles are approached straight, and others curved.

This is very beneficial for the pelvic muscles, the back and abdominals and the thoracic sling in the front end of the horse.

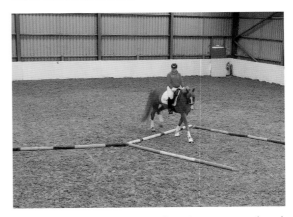

In the walk, the horse is performing an acute bend and is well positioned to achieve this.

The Half Moon: This exercise requires five poles positioned on the ground in a half-moon configuration. The horse is ridden over the outside poles, gradually working inside where the exercise becomes more difficult. The horse should take three steps between the outside poles and one single step between the inner side poles. The horse continues in this sequence and then changes direction.

This is very beneficial for strengthening the trunk and shoulder muscles.

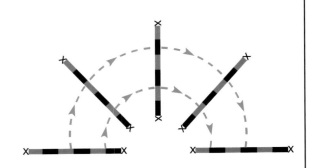

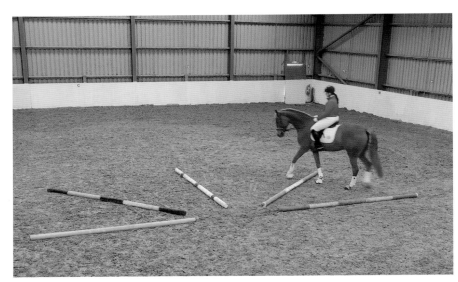

Walking over the outer edge of the half moon ground poles. The horse is moving nicely on the bit and in good balance.

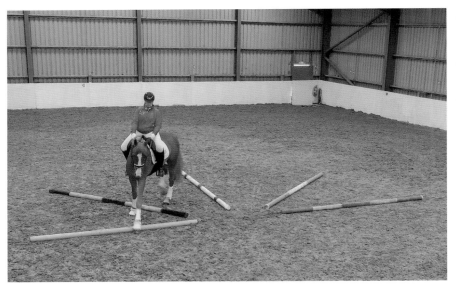

Walking over the inner edge of the half moon ground poles. The horse is bending nicely, maximising the use of its body.

Randomly Scattered Poles: There are numerous options available when riding randomly scattered poles: you can ride around, between and over the poles, performing different shapes. You can walk or trot over the poles and perform half halts in front of some. Performed in walk, trot or canter. A combination of gaits is excellent for the horse's focus and varies the intensity of the exercise.

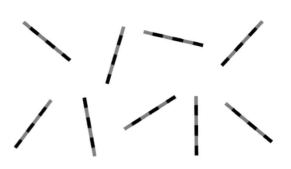

This exercise requires anything from six to nine poles placed randomly in the arena on the ground, but the occasional cavaletti could be included.

Very beneficial for proprioception and all the deep postural and superficial muscles.

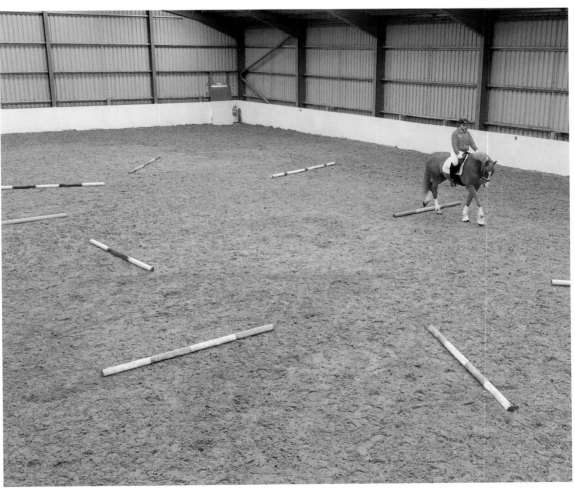

The walking portion of the randomly scattered poles. The horse is thinking and focusing on its foot placement.

The Four Star: This exercise can be performed in either walk or trot, following a circular path around the outside of the poles or by traversing the edge of the pole in a square shape. As you progress, gradually decrease the size of the circle. The objective is to maintain control over the horse's shoulders to prevent excessive swinging of the hindquarters. Strive for a balanced position where the hindquarters neither swing out too far nor too far in, achieving harmonious coordination between the shoulders and hindquarters.

This exercise requires four poles to be set in a star pattern on the ground. Very beneficial for the neck, shoulder, back and abdominal muscles.

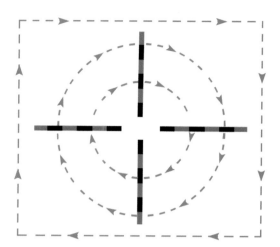

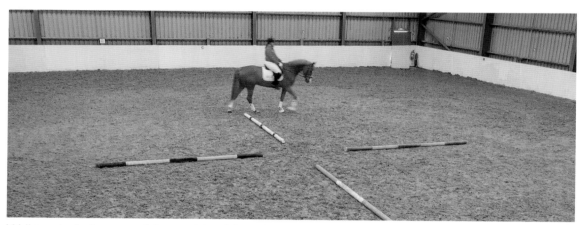

Walking clockwise around the outside of the poles in a circle the horse is nicely balanced and on the bit.

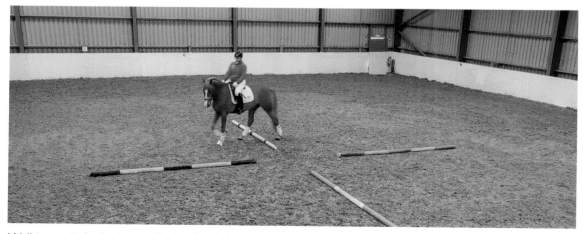

Walking anti-clockwise on the inside of the poles in a circle, the horse is bending nicely.

Four Square: This exercise involves riding in a straight line around the outside of the square formed by the poles, making a turn as you navigate the corners. Riding on the outside of the square represents a lower difficulty level than on the inside.

This exercise requires four poles to be set in a large square. Very beneficial for the neck, shoulder, back, abdominal and hindquarter muscles.

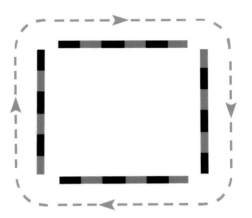

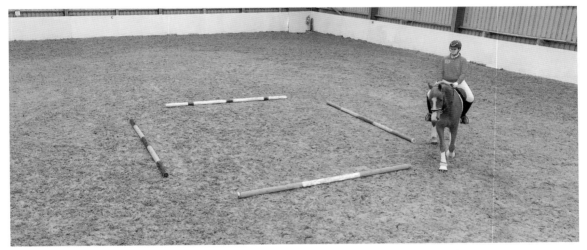

Walking clockwise around the outside of the square poles, creating a nice bend at the corner.

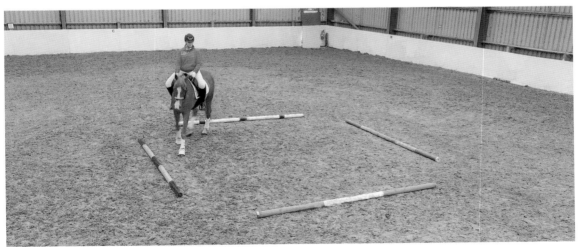

Walking anti-clockwise around the inside of the square poles, creating a nice acute bend.

Gymnastic Exercises

Incorporating gymnastic pole work into the training performed in trot and canter can be very beneficial for the horse, such as:

- Develops strength, condition and coordination by requiring the horse to use its body differently. These exercises challenge the horse to maintain balance and control their movements, which can improve their overall athleticism and fitness.
- Increases flexibility, which encourages the horse to stretch and reach for the poles, which can help to increase range of motion. This can be particularly beneficial for horses that have tight or stiff muscles and need to lengthen them through movement.
- Enhances proprioception abilities by challenging them to adjust their body position and stride to navigate the poles.
- Builds confidence in its abilities, as the horse becomes more comfortable navigating the poles, it may feel more confident in its movements, which can translate to other aspects of its training.
- Improves jumping technique, hence very beneficial for horses that are being trained for jumping. It helps with its take-off and landing positions, as well as the ability to adjust its stride between jumps.

Gymnastic Cavaletti Serpentine: This exercise requires three cavaletti poles to be set across the centre line, as wide apart as possible so the horse can use the entire area. The poles are ridden in a serpentine style in trot first, then canter and changing the lead through the sequence.

Very beneficial for general strength, conditioning and co-ordination, proprioception, focus and balance.

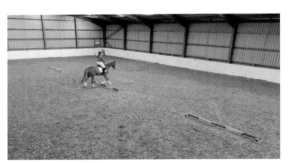

Trotting over the centre raised pole at a nice even pace.

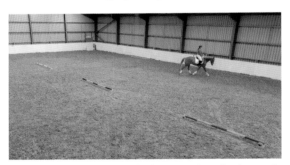

Taking a deep right bend, showing that the horse is on the bit and moving nicely in engagement.

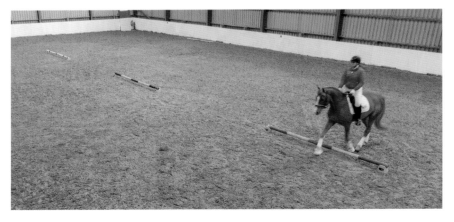

Trotting over the final raised pole, the horse and rider focused and looking ahead.

Gymnastic Cavaletti Free Style: The sequence is ridden by approaching the single cavaletti then over a bounce, sweeping around on a bend, then over another bounce riding straight to the next single cavaletti, then repeat as necessary or varying the route you take.

This exercise requires six raised poles set around the arena. Very beneficial for general strength, conditioning and co-ordination, proprioception, focus and balance.

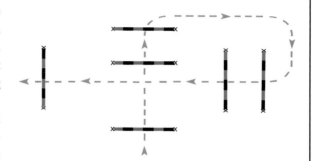

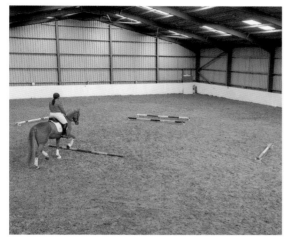

Trotting over a single cavaletti, the horse is nicely picking up its front limbs.

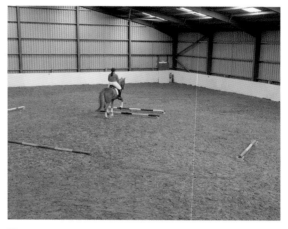

Trotting over a bounce before completing a turn to the right. The image gives a sense of distance and good use of the arena.

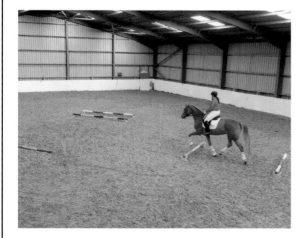

Trotting over a bounce. The horse is looking forward and thinking about the next pole.

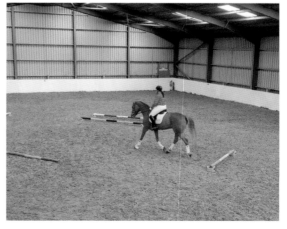

Heading towards a cavaletti to complete the sequence, the horse is on the bit, engaged and tracking up throughout.

Gymnastic Grid: The sequence is set up as four trotting poles, two cross-pole jumps (bounces) and one final vertical jump. This is ridden in trot and canter depending on the horse's fitness. If the horse struggles with this exercise, return to some more basic ones.

Very beneficial for general strength, conditioning and co-ordination, proprioception, focus and balance.

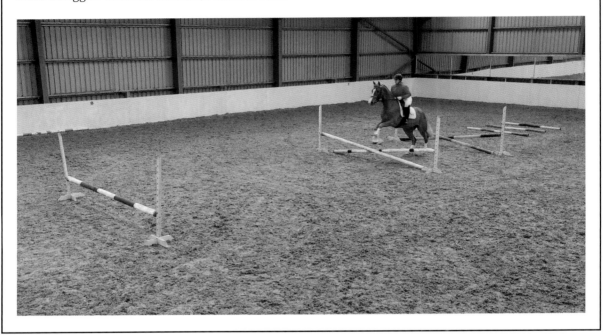

★ TOP TIP

To perform these exercises in the best possible way, the horse should be warmed up and moving in balance. The rider should be balanced with proper body position and stability throughout all exercises, with their eyes up and using subtle cues to communicate with the horse.

The horse should enter any pole pattern at a controlled speed, walk, trot or canter guided by the rider. The horse should be ready to make timely and precise transitions between poles, direction changes, etc., following the rider's cues.

Timing and coordination are very important: the horse and rider must work together to maintain the correct path and timing. This involves precise steering, balance and coordination to avoid knocking poles or deviating from the planned pole work pattern.

If the horse or rider is struggling whatsoever, then do not progress to a more challenging exercise until the basics are mastered. This will not be beneficial for you or your horse and will hinder the progression.

Find pleasure in diversifying your horse's routine, and experimenting with different activities each week. This approach not only keeps both you and your horse engaged but also alleviates monotony. Remember that it is essential to strike a balance between difficulty and intensity, as overwhelming your horse with excessive mental stimulation or physical activity should be avoided.

Conclusion

Throughout this book, we have explored the realms of developing our equine understanding, enhancing our management, providing manual therapy and adopting correct supportive exercise. We are left with a profound understanding of the impact these practices can have on the wellbeing and performance of our horses. We have also discovered that by combining science, intuition and compassionate care, we can unlock the true potential that lies within each horse.

Equine management encompasses an holistic approach to caring for our horses, acknowledging their physical, mental and emotional needs. From proper nutrition and a suitable environment to regular tack checks and attention to their social dynamics, we have learned that every aspect of their wellbeing matters. By nurturing a harmonious and balanced lifestyle, we lay the foundation for optimal health and wellness.

The integration of manual therapy has illuminated a new path in equine care, allowing us to understand and address the subtleties of their bodies. Through the power of touch, we can detect tension, release it and restore balance to their musculoskeletal system. Manual therapy techniques offer us the ability to alleviate pain, promote relaxation and enhance overall function. By embracing these techniques, we become partners in our horses' physical well-being, aiding them in reaching their full potential.

Furthermore, by implementing exercises that are tailored to the individual needs of each horse, we can enhance their strength, flexibility and coordination. From groundwork to under-saddle exercises, we have explored the importance of engaging the horse's body and mind in a progressive manner. Through a systematic approach, we can develop their musculature, improve their balance and refine their performance. By building a solid foundation through manual therapy and correct supportive exercise, we create a platform for the horse to excel in their chosen discipline.

As we close the final chapter of this book, let us carry forward the knowledge we have gained and embrace the responsibility that comes with our passion for horses. May we remain steadfast in our pursuit of understanding, always striving to deepen our connection with these magnificent animals. Let us remember that equine management, manual therapy and correct supportive exercise are not merely tools but vehicles that guide us towards a world in which horses thrive.

Together, let us be advocates for our horses, empowering them to be the best versions of themselves. Through our unwavering dedication and the application of the knowledge shared within these pages, we can shape a future in which every horse experiences a life filled with respect, good health, vitality, love and happiness.

Acknowledgements

I would like to express my deepest gratitude to the numerous people who have played an indispensable role in my equine journey. Although their contributions are too vast to mention comprehensively, I would like to take a moment to extend my heartfelt appreciation to some of them.

Firstly, I am immensely grateful to Sally Spencer, whose unwavering encouragement inspired me to break free from my corporate career and embark on this transformative journey with horses. Your support and belief in me have been invaluable.

I extend my sincere thanks to Millicent Sword, not only for proofreading sections of this book but also for her assistance in sourcing meaningful photography: your attention to detail and unwavering dedication have significantly enhanced the quality of this work. I would also like to express my gratitude to Marie Stephenson, Therese Murphy, Donna Barker and again, Millicent Sword, my colleagues, whose unwavering support in my professional endeavours has given me the necessary time and space to dedicate to the writing of this book.

A special mention goes to Emma Sheridan, an exceptional photographer whose remarkable skills captured the essence of this book through countless hours of braving the elements, whether it be wind, rain, or rare moments of sunshine. Your dedication and artistry have brought the pages of this book to life.

I am deeply indebted to Stephanie Easterby, whose horse After Eight patiently posed for the many manual therapy photographs. Belinda Waites and Esme, Christine Andrea Bunting and Puddle, Amanda Jane Brawn and Paddy, Laura Frisby and Faramir, Laura Kenyon-Brodie and Maisie, Rebecca Brusby and Bentley, Joanna Rawson and Twinshock DD – each of them played a role in preparing their lovely horses for photographs. Lizzie Hill and the lovely Eddie, who rode in some beautiful styles so I could explain gait, and Amy Lauren Fillingham who played a crucial role when capturing the correct supportive exercises under the drone with her delightful horse, Rocky. Your participation and expertise have greatly enriched the content of this book.

A thank you goes to Deanna Montero, whose illustrations have added a unique visual dimension to this work.

To my Mother Jessie, whose love, patience, support and understanding have been invaluable, not only during the writing process but throughout my entire life.

Lastly, I would like to express my heartfelt gratitude to my husband, Mark. Your unwavering support, provision of captivating imagery for this book, and understanding of the countless hours I spent at my computer writing it have been indispensable. Your love and encouragement have fuelled my passion and dedication throughout this journey.

To all those who have contributed to this book, whether mentioned here or not, I extend my deepest thanks; your presence and support have shaped this work in immeasurable ways, and for that, I am forever grateful.

Love always to my missing companions, Shamus and Joe. Long may your spirits roam free in the realm of equine grace, and thank you for the indelible imprint you left on my soul.

Bibliography

Aristotle Ballou, **J.**, *55 Corrective Exercises for Horses* (Trafalgar Square Books, 2018)

Beckstett, A., 'Rein-Lameness Associated With TMJ Pain in Horses' *https://thehorse.com/1119428/rein-lameness-associated-with-tmj-pain-in-horses/* (accessed 11 January 2023)

Blocksdorf, K., 'A Picture Guide to the Different Parts of a Horse' *https://www.thesprucepets.com/the-parts-of-a-horse-1887388* (accessed 10 January 2023)

Calzone, S., Wilkins, C., Deckers, I., and Nankervis, K. (2022) 'The Effects of the EquiAmiTM Training Aid on the Kinematics of the Horse at the Walk and Trot In-Hand' *Journal of Equine Veterinary Science* 111 *https://doi.org/10.1016/j.jevs.2022.103868.* (accessed 15 January 2023)

Colborne, G.R., Tang, L., Adams, B., Gordon, B., McCabe, B., and Riley, C. (2021) 'A Novel Load Cell-Supported Research Platform to Measure Vertical and Horizontal Motion of a Horse's Centre of Mass During Trailer Transport' *Journal of Equine Veterinary Science* 99 *https://doi.org/10.1016/j.jevs.2021.103408* (accessed 10 January 2023)

Dalla Costa, E., Minero, M., Lebelt, D., Stucke, D., Canali, E., and Leach, M.C. (2014) 'Development of the Horse Grimace Scale (HGS) as a pain assessment tool in horses undergoing routine castration'. *PLoS One.* *https://www.ncbi.nlm.nih.gov/pmc/articles/PMC3960217/* (accessed 18 January 2023)

Deep Recover (2014) 'The benefits of sports massage' *https://deeprecovery.com/sports-massage-benefits-for-athletes/* (accessed 10 January 2023)

Dockalova, H., Baholet, D., Batik, A., Zeman, L., and Horky, P. (2022) 'Effect of Milk Thistle (Silybum marianum) Seed Cakes by Horses Subjected to Physical Exertion'. *Journal of Equine Vet Science* *https://pubmed.ncbi.nlm.nih.gov/35318098/* (accessed 10 January 2023)

Dyson, S., Berger, J., Ellis, A., and Mullard, J. (2017) 'Can the presence of musculoskeletal pain be determined from the facial expressions of ridden horses (FEReq)?' *Journal of Veterinary Behaviour* 19 pp. 78–89, *https://doi.org/10.1016/j.jveb.2017.03.005* (accessed 10 February 2023)

Hill, C., and Crook, T. (2010) 'The relationship between massage to the equine caudal hindlimb muscles and hindlimb protraction'. *Equine Veterinary Journal*, 42 pp. 683–687 *https://doi.org/10.1111/j.2042-3306.2010.00279* (accessed 10 January 2023)

Horses and Us (2023) 'The 4 Basic Horse Gaits Explained [Diagrams & Animations]' *https://www.horsesandus.com/the-4-basic-horse-gaits-explained/* (accessed 13 January 2023)

Impact Physical Therapy (2023) 'Benefits of Massage Therapy for Athletes' *https://www.impactphysicaltherapy.com/benefits-massage-therapy-athletes/* (accessed 10 January 2023)

J.W. Equine (2023) 'An Introduction to Functional Conformation' *https://hcbc.ca/wp-content/uploads/2021/11/2021-An-Introduction-to-Functional-Conformation.pdf* (accessed 10 January 2023)

Lilley, C., *Schooling with Ground Poles: Flatwork Schooling for Every Horse and Rider* (J.A.Allen & Co Ltd, 2003)

McMaster University (2012) 'Massage is promising for muscle recovery: McMaster researchers find 10 minutes reduces inflammation' *https://www.mcmaster.ca/opr/html/opr/media/main/NewsReleases/MassageispromisingformusclerecoveryMcMasterresearchersfind10minutesreducesinflammation.htm* (accessed 20 March 2023)

Medical Massage Therapy (2023) 'The effects of massage therapy' *https://www.massagetherapyreference.com/effects-of-massage-therapy/* (accessed 20 March 2023)

Raspa, F., Roggero, A., Palestrini, C., Marten Canavesio, M., Bergero, D., and Valle, E. (2021) 'Studying the Shape Variations of the Back, the Neck, and the Mandibular Angle of Horses Depending on Specific Feeding Postures Using Geometric Morphometrics'. *Animals* 11 p. 763. : *https://doi.org/10.3390/ani11030763* (accessed 20 March 2023)

Sarah Warne (2013) 'Classical training, letting go of the ego and excuses' *https://www.eurodressage.com/2013/02/25/classical-training-letting-go-ego-and-excuses* (accessed 22 March 2023)

Wikipedia (2023) 'Horse Teeth' *https://en.wikipedia.org/wiki/Horse_teeth* (accessed 24 March 2023)

Zaneb, H., Peham, C., and Stanek, C. (2013) 'Functional anatomy and biomechanics of the equine thoracolumbar spine: a review' *Turkish Journal of Veterinary & Animal Sciences:* 37 *https://doi.org/10.3906/vet-1205-45* (accessed 20 February 2023)

Index

First published in 2024 by J.A. Allen,
an imprint of The Crowood Press Ltd,
Ramsbury, Marlborough Wiltshire SN8 2HR

enquiries@crowood.com

www.crowood.com

British Library Cataloguing-in-Publication Data
A catalogue record for this book is available
from the British Library.

ISBN: 978 0 7198 3507 0

Typeset by surichardsgraphicdesign.com

Printed and bound in India by Replika Press Pvt Ltd